PALEO DIET COOKBOOK

Delicious Recipes to Lose Weight and Achieve a Healthy Lifestyle

(The Ultimate Beginner's Guide to Paleo Diet Plan)

I0222624

Mildred Oshea

Published by Alex Howard

Mildred Oshea

Paleo Diet Cookbook: Delicious Recipes to Lose Weight and Achieve a Healthy Lifestyle (The Ultimate Beginner's Guide to Paleo Diet Plan)

ISBN 978-1-77485-028-2

Legal & Disclaimer

The information contained in this book is not designed to replace or take the place of any form of medicine or professional medical advice. The information in this book has been provided for educational and entertainment purposes only.

The information contained in this book has been compiled from sources deemed reliable, and it is accurate to the best of the Author's knowledge; however, the Author cannot guarantee its accuracy and validity and cannot be held liable for any errors or omissions. Changes are periodically made to this book. You must consult your doctor or get professional medical advice before using any of the suggested remedies, techniques, or information in this book.

Upon using the information contained in this book, you agree to hold harmless the Author from and against any damages, costs, and expenses, including any legal fees potentially resulting from the application of any of the information provided by this guide. This disclaimer applies to any damages or injury caused by the use and application, whether directly or indirectly, of any advice or information presented, whether for breach of contract, tort, negligence, personal injury, criminal intent, or under any other cause of action.

Table of Contents

Part 1

Introduction

Paleo diet aka caveman diet is famous for the consumption of plants and animals. People eat diet just like people eaten during the Paleolithic era. Numerous experiments show that if you follow a paleo diet, then you can automatically decrease the chances of acquiring disease just because of the food. The Paleo diet was first time introduced in the 1960s, but it was failed to get the attention of people. In 1975, people started noticing it because it is about food and eating habits of your ancestors. Following a Paleo diet doesn't mean to live in caves, hunt for food and live without modern amenities. It is all about food instead of a lifestyle and you can follow this diet to get lots of health benefits.

There are various versions of Paleo diet, but all follow three creeds, such as:

- Food collected by hunters
- Large amounts of non-starchy veggies
- Consumption of grass fed lean protein

Some Paleo eaters are also allowed to consume fruits and nuts except peanuts because these fall in the category of legumes. You have to include raw and clean food in your diet while dumping grains, legumes, sugar, dairy and processed food. The omega-3 fats, olive oil, coconut oil and vegetable oils are allowed, but the refined oils are prohibited. You have to eat real food, such as the food that you can hunt and grow, despite starchy vegetables.

The Paleo diet is particularly designed to avoid the worst effects of overly-processed and carbohydrate food. The western diet is not good for your health because you may suffer from lots of chronic diseases. The type 2 diabetes, cancer and cardiovascular diseases are common with the consumption of processed food. The processed food promotes obesity and digestive issues and creates havoc in your life. The Paleo diet is a good step toward a healthy body because the real food will save you from lots of health problems.

This book is designed as a guide for you so that you can learn about Paleo diet, meal plans. Exercise programs and common mistakes. If you want to follow a Paleo diet, then this book will be a good start for you.

Chapter 1: What Is Paleo Diet? Benefits Of Paleo Diet

The Paleolithic diet is simple and straightforward because it requires you to get rid of processed and high-carb food. You will follow the diet of a caveman while avoiding lectins and gluten. You need to eat natural food and avoid all types of processed and unhealthy food. High consumption of processed food, gluten and carbohydrates may lead you to obesity, cancer, diabetes and reproductive problems. People often misunderstand Paleo diet and try to avoid it, but, in fact, it is a beneficial diet. It is all about food because people often misunderstand that it means to follow a caveman lifestyle. You have to change your eating habits and stick to real food.

Benefits of Paleo Diet

The Paleo diet is a healthy way to eat and avoid lots of health problems. It can keep you lean, strong and energetic while reducing the threat of diabetes, heart diseases, cancer, obesity, and infertility. You have to avoid a modern diet that is full of refined foods, sugar and trans fats. There are some benefits of Paleo Diet that will help you to understand how this diet is good for your health:

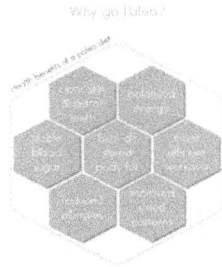

Get Healthy Cells

The human body cells are made of saturated and unsaturated fat and the composition of your cell is based on a healthy diet. The paleo diet can naturally balance your body fat by limiting the consumption of unhealthy food. The Omega-3 fatty acids play an important role to enhance the performance of the brain and promote better growth and development.

Healthy Brain

The Paleo diet enables you to get protein and fat from healthy sources, such as salmon. The salmon is packed with omega 3 fatty acids and it is the main content lacking in the diet of an average man. The Omega 3 fatty acids are good for your body because DHA plays an active role in the health of the eyes, heart, and brain.

Increase Muscle and Reduce Fat

Paleo diet is based on animal meat and it is a healthy source of protein. The anabolic protein is used to build new cells and it will increase your muscle mass. The more muscles will increase your metabolism rate and you will get more energy to move bigger muscles. It proves helpful for the body to send energy to muscle cells instead of fat cells. An increase in the muscle cells will automatically reduce the fat cells. The healthy paleo diet will help your body to increase the energy to transport to glycogen in your muscles instead of triglycerides found in fat cells. Muscles require more energy than fat and with a higher percentage of muscle than fat, you may have a higher BMR.

Better Gut Health

The sugar and processed food can increase your body fat and cause inflammation in your intestinal tract. The processed food can be the reason of stress because it may cause leaky gut syndrome. If you want to avoid problems with the digestive tract, then you should follow Paleo diet. The bolus of blood sugar with meals and refined carbohydrates, such as white bread, white rice, and sugar loaded soda can increase the levels of cytokines also known as an inflammatory messenger.

Circle of Life

The Paleo diet promotes the consumption of meats and eggs raised on pasture. The animals should be raised naturally on grass for their entire life. The cows and chickens should roam together in the meadow for better synergy. In the natural environment, the chickens eat larvae and bugs found under the cow pies. The cow pie can be a great fertilizer for the grass and it will provide food to the cows. The natural diet is great for animals because this food is loaded with nutrients and these animals will be healthy for your diet. The eggs and meat raised in a pasture contain 10 times more omega3s than the factory hens and eggs.

Lots of Vitamins and Minerals

You can eat a variety of vegetables and fruits of different colors. To get better health, it will be good to make your plate colorful by including a variety of vegetables and fruits of the season. The colors of the vegetables reflect the presence of particular nutrients. You can eat rainbow to get all your vitamins.

Limit Fructose

The human body reacts differently to digest fructose than other carbohydrates. The Paleo diet suggests the limited consumption of fructose; therefore, you have to be very careful while selecting fruit. You should avoid banana and include Kiwi in your diet. It is good to limit your diet to 2 to 3 pieces of fruit on a regular basis.

Digestion and Absorption

The paleo diet will increase your ability to digest and absorb food because the grass-fed beef is better than factory raised meat. A strict paleo diet for 30 days is good to solve your digestion problems. You will feel better after 30 days because the paleo diet can solve lots of digestion and absorption problems. Food items consumed in the paleo diet can help you to get rid of allergies and additional body fat.

Good for Allergies and Inflammation

The paleo diet will help you to reduce the consumption of allergens, such as grains. After reducing the consumption of grains, you can get rid of lots of allergies. It is good for inflammation and cardiovascular diseases because this diet focuses on Omega 3 fatty acids. The animals raised in the meadow have a better ratio of omega 3 and 6.

Better to Reduce Weight

The Paleo diet will help you to reduce weight and get more energy by reducing the consumption of sugar, coffee, and unhealthy fat. The paleo diet aka low carb diet is good for your health because after removing processed foods, you can drastically reduce additional pounds. You can increase your insulin sensitivity because sugary foods are not good for your health. It will reduce the risk of various diseases and shrink fat cells.

Chapter 2: Foods That You Eat During Paleo Diet And Foods To Avoid

In order to follow a Paleo diet, you have to avoid consumption of particular food items. You should be careful with the food that you can eat or avoid:

EAT	DON'T EAT
Meadow-raised meats	Cereal grains
Sea food	Legumes (peanuts as well)
Naturally grown fruits and veggies	Processed foods
Eggs	Refined sugar
Nuts and seeds	Potatoes
Healthy oils (Olive, coconut, flax seeds and walnut)	Dairy
	Salt
	Refined oils

Tips to Build a Healthy Paleo Diet

There are some tips that will help you to build a healthy paleo diet because there are some foods that should be included in your diet:

Lean Proteins

Lean proteins are important for strong muscles, healthy bones, and best possible immune function. The protein will increase your satisfaction level and reduce your craving for unhealthy foods.

Fruits and Vegetables

The fruits and vegetables are good for your health because these are rich in vitamins, mineral, antioxidants and phytonutrients. Consumption of fruits and vegetables can increase the chances diabetes, cancer, and neurological problems.

Healthy Fats

You should consume healthy fat obtained from nuts, avocados, seeds, fish oil, olive and grass-fed meat. The Omega-3 and monosaturated fats will help you to reduce the chances of cancer, diabetes, cardiovascular disease and obesity.

Paleo Diet Routine

The Paleo diet is based on the unprocessed foods because this diet is good to avoid obesity, diabetes, and cardiovascular diseases. There is no right way to eat food, but you have to focus on the healthy foods and avoid dairy, grains, legumes, soybean, sunflower, corn and grape seed oil. There is a sample diet routine that will help you to follow a paleo diet:

Paleo Breakfast

At the breakfast, you can make an omelet with broccoli, mushrooms, and onion. Make sure to use olive oil, omega-3 enriched food and slices of chicken breast.

Paleo Lunches

In the initial week, you can enjoy a salad with mixed greens, radishes, spinach, bell peppers, carrots, cucumber, almonds, avocados, walnuts, apples, pears, etc. The salads can be prepared with the combination of different vegetables, nuts, and fruits. You can use olive oil and black pepper to enhance the flavor or your salad. Lemon juice is important to reduce body fat. You can mix pieces of chicken, beef, turkey or lamb. Seafood is a good choice, such as salmon, tuna, seafood, etc.

Paleo Dinner

In the dinner, you can try spaghetti squash with pasta that should be topped with marinara and pesto. Roasted beet and chicken will be a great dinner with steamed broccoli, spinach, and steamed asparagus. Salmon, tuna, and halibut are great to grill with olive oil and garlic. Your dinner should be packed with vegetables and lean meat to get lots of proteins.

Pale Desserts

You can get the advantage of berries and other succulent fruits because it is great for dessert. The carrot, celery stick and slices of fruits are great to satisfy your dessert cravings.

Sample Breakfast:

• Breakfast: Omega-3 or scrambled eggs cooked in olive oil with fresh parsley. You should take one glass of Grapefruit or other fresh fruit juice. A cup of herbal tea will be good for your health.

• Snack: Sliced lean beef, fresh apricots or seasonal fruit

• Lunch: Enjoy salad with chicken, olive oil and lemon juice. You need a cup of herbal tea to reduce weight.

- Snack: In snacks, you can enjoy slices of apple and raw walnuts.

- Dinner: At dinner, you can take a few avocado and tomato slices, grilled chicken breast, baked broccoli, artichoke, carrots and a bowl of berries, almond, and raisins. You need one glass of mineral water and as per rule, you are allowed to consume three non-Paleo meals in each week

Chapter 3: Paleo Shopping List And 14 Day Meal Plan

If you want to follow a paleo meal, it is important to have all relevant ingredients in your pantry. There is a sample shopping list that will help you to get an idea for Paleo shopping:

You need to buy whole foods and it will be better to visit the farmer's market for the fresh fruits, vegetables, meats and other important items.

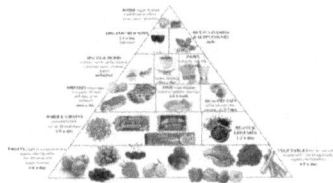

Buy Lean Meats

There are 10 essential animal proteins that should be unprocessed and free from hormone and antibiotic. The animals should be naturally raised in the meadow:

- Beef, Bison, and Buffalo
- Chicken, Turkey, and Duck (Free from skin and fat)
- Eggs
- Game Meats (Venison, Rabbit, Wild Boar)
- Lamb and Goat
- Kidneys, sweetbreads, tongue, livers and marrow organs

Sea Food

You can buy Paleo-friendly seafood because it has lots of protein and Omega fats to promote weight loss:

- Cod
- Anchovies
- Flounder
- Bass
- Halibut
- Salmon
- Mahi Mahi
- Shellfish (mussels, shrimp, crab, lobster and scallops)
- Sardines
- Tuna

Paleo Fruits

There are lots of fruits that are allowed in the Paleo diet, but you should avoid high sugar food. There are some simple guidelines for the selection of fruits in the Paleo diet:

Limit the Consumption of High-sugar Fruits

Your diet should not include banana, mangoes, pineapple, dates and watermelon. You should avoid them if you are trying to reduce weight.

Dried Fruits

You can consume moderate amounts of dried fruits, such as mix one spoon in the salad to use as snacks. The nuts should be free from excessive sugar and salt because these can increase your calorie intake. You should consume in moderation because high consumption of dried fruit is not good for your health.

Avocados are Important

The Avocados have the healthy fats and you should include them in your diet.

Paleo Vegetables

Just like fruits, you can consume almost every vegetable, but be careful with starchy tubers. There are two notable things about the shopping of vegetables:

• Starchy Tubers: You should limit the consumption of potatoes and sweet potatoes because their excessive amounts are not good.

• Legumes: Chickpeas, peas, soybeans, and lentils are not good to take in Paleo diet because you should remove them from your list.

Nuts and Seeds

Nuts and seeds are famous for using as snacks in the paleo diet and these are great to give a crunchy touch to your recipes. Make sure to have them without any added salt, sugar, and unhealthy fat. You are not allowed to take peanuts because these are also considered a form of legume.

• Good Nuts for Paleo Diet: Cashews, Almonds, Macadamia Nuts, Walnuts, Pecans, Pistachios, etc.

• Good Seeds for Paleo Diet: Pumpkin, Sunflower, Sesame, Flaxseeds.

Healthy Oils

Healthy oils are important for health, but in Paleo diet, you can't use vegetable oil, canola and peanut oil. Highly refined oils are not good for your health because these have a high concentration of polyunsaturated omega 6 fatty acids that can be the reason of inflammation in your body. You need oil with high omega-3 that can reduce inflammation. Try to buy paleo approved oils that are available in the most unprocessed form, such as extra-virgin olive oil.

• To use as salad dressings, you can use avocado oil. It is also good to cook food on a low heat.

• Coconut oil is good for all kinds of cooking.

• Flaxseed oils are excellent to use as omega 3 supplements.

• Extra-virgin olive oil is good to use in salad, cooking, and frying.

• Sesame oil will be seasoned on the cooked food.

• You can use small amounts of walnut oil in salads.

Healthy Beverages

If you want to include healthy beverages in your diet, then pick fresh juices and flavored milk without high sugar concentration. You can the following beverages:

• Coffee and tea without sugar and milk

• Soda water

• Coconut water

• Almond milk

• Plain Water

• Soda water

- Coconut milk

Sweets and Treats for Paleo Diet

You can take a limited amount of alcohol in the Paleo diet, but make it an occasional treat only. The dark chocolate is good for your heart and you can add unprocessed honey to your meals to make them sweet. Coconut products and stevia are also good to take as zero calorie sweeteners.

Sample Meals Plan of 14 Days

Meal Plan for First Week:

Breakfast	Lunch	Dinner	Snack
One bowl of berries and coconut milk	Roasted chicken with cherry tomatoes and salad. You can sprinkle olive oil and lemon juice.	Special Paleo Spaghetti	One tablespoon Macadamia nuts
Surplus paleo spaghetti	Chicken and vegetable soup	Beef goulash (try any paleo recipe)	Beef jerky
Omelete of onion and spinach	Tuna salad with lettuce and almonds	Grilled trout and squash soup	Boiled eggs (hard)
		Coconut ice cream as dessert	

Chicken and eggs with a few slices of fruit	Zucchini and sweet potato	Beef bourguignon	Chicken slices
Coconut milk	Citrus salad of beef	Citrus baked chicken	Berries and almonds (one bowl)
Cold chicken roast with mayo	Scallops with lemon and garlic	Waldorf salad	Bacon covered with dark chocolate
	Coconut ice cream, enjoy as dessert	Baked apples to enjoy as dessert	
Fried eggs and tomatoes	Salad of broccoli and grapes	Butter chicken	Raw vegetables

Meal Plan for Second Week

18

Breakfast	Lunch	Dinner	Snack
Paleo cereal: Special cereal with nuts and berries. Make sure to add coconut milk.			
Egg salad with lettuce	Roast beef with vegetables	Plantain chips	
Roasted beef slices and pesto	Beef and cabbage poach	Mustard pork haunch with coleslaw	Coconut ice cream dessert
Pork sausages and grapefruit	Minced beef in bell peppers	Duck confit with carrot	One can of salmon with olive oil and lime juice
Eggs with salsa	Coconut curry (stir fry)	Paleo Shepherd's pie (use cauliflower instead of potatoes)	Smoked tuna
Fried beef minced and carrots	Bacon, boiled eggs and tomato with low fat mayo	Polish stew	Peppery pumpkin seeds
Chicken and asparagus omelet	Mussels and garlic sauce	Chicken with olive, garlic and lemon	
Dessert: Poached Pears	Celery sticks		
Beef liver and baked broccoli with	Fried lamb chops and cooked	Pumpkin Chili	Olives and sauerkraut

salsa	spinach		

Paleo Exercises

You can take the advantage of modern equipment because to some exercises are important to follow to reduce your weight. The caveman exercises are broken down into following movements:

- Bending
- Lunging
- Squatting
- Pushing
- Twisting
- Pulling
- Running
- Gait-related exercising (30 Seconds)

You can do these exercises to melt your body fat and get lots of other health benefits.

Chapter 4: Good Paleo Diet Recipes

There are some Paleo diet recipes that you can try during your paleo diet and avoid consumption of unhealthy food items:

Recipe 01: Scrambled Eggs

- 4 slices raw chicken
- 6 eggs
- 1 teaspoon radish

Directions:

Take a cooking pan and snip chicken into a skillet with kitchen shears. Saute it to make crispy. Beat eggs with radish and pour eggs in the greased cooking pan. Scramble eggs and add crispy chicken pieces to mix them.

Recipe 02: Menemen Breakfast

- ¼ chopped onion, red
- 1 diced tomato
- ½ cup bell pepper, chopped
- 1 tablespoon olive oil
- ¼ teaspoon red-pepper flakes
- 1 chopped garlic clove
- ¼ teaspoon cumin powder
- ¼ teaspoon ground black pepper

- ¼ teaspoon turmeric powder
- ¼ teaspoon salt
- 3 eggs
- 1 tablespoon parsley, chopped

Directions:

Take a big pan and cook onion, pepper and tomato on the low heat. Chop garlic and add to the skillet along with spices. Now add vegetables and cook to tender them. While cooking vegetables, you can beat eggs. Add sauce in the pan with eggs to scramble them. When they become creamy, remove to serve on a plate and sprinkle parsley.

Recipe 03: Guacamole For Lunch

- 2 tablespoons crushed onion
- 1 garlic clove, chopped
- 2 avocados (halved)
- ½ lime
- Hot sauce as per taste
- Salt as per taste
- 1 tablespoon chopped cilantro

Directions:

Remove the flesh of avocados in a bowl, mix onion and garlic. Mash up this mixture and squeeze lime on it and then add hot sauce. Add salt and cilantro to blend this mixture with a fork. You can serve it immediately.

Recipe 04: Tuna Salad

- 2 cups lettuce leaves, chopped
- 1/4 cup basil
- 1/2 cup cherry tomatoes, chopped
- 1/4 red onion, chopped
- 8-ounce tuna steak
- 2 cucumbers, crosswise slices
- 4 radishes, thin sliced
- 2 hard-boiled eggs, chopped
- 2 teaspoons capers
- Olive oil for cooking
- 1 teaspoon mustard
- 1/4 teaspoon maple syrup
- 1/4 teaspoon kosher salt
- Fresh cracked black pepper
- 1 tablespoon lemon juice
- 1 teaspoon water
- 1/2 garlic clove, chopped
- 1 tablespoon olive oil (extra-virgin)

Directions:

Take a plate to arrange eggs, radishes, cucumbers, tomatoes, basil, onion and lettuce. Take a pan after greasing it with cooking spray and add tuna after sprinkling salt and pepper. Cook tuna on each side and then arrange tuna on vegetables.

Prepare the dressing by blending lemon juice and remaining ingredients in a small jar with tight lid. Shake well to combine the sauce and sprinkle on the salads.

Recipe 05: Zucchini And Cauliflower Frittata

- 2 tablespoons butter or coconut oil
- 1 large cauliflower, chopped
- 2 zucchinis, chopped
- 2 tablespoons parsley
- Salt and pepper as per taste
- 8 eggs
- 1 Red bell pepper, chopped

Directions:

Cook chopped cauliflower in a cooking pan on medium heat for four minutes and then add bell pepper and zucchini slices. It will take eight minutes to cook. Beat eggs in a bowl and mix salt and pepper. Now pour this mixture on vegetables and cook on a low heat for 10 minutes. Finish cooking when it becomes golden and serve with fresh parsley.

Recipe 06: Turkey Chili

- 3 to 4 cups turkey
- 2 cups chopped carrots
- 2 cups sliced tomatoes
- 2 cups chopped onions
- 2 chopped bell pepper
- 1 tablespoon flakes of red chili

- 2 tablespoons tomato paste
- 4 garlic cloves, crushed
- 1 cup chicken stock
- 2 tablespoons chili powder
- 1 tablespoon cumin powder
- Sea salt and black pepper powder to taste;
- 1 tablespoon oregano
- Paleo fat for cooking
- Green onions, chopped (garnish)

Directions:

Melt some fat in a large skillet and then add peppers, onions, and carrots to cook for five minutes. It is time to sprinkle, red pepper, chili powder, garlic, cumin, and oregano. Mix them well and cook for one minute.

Now transfer tomatoes, stock, tomato paste, and meat. Sprinkle salt and pepper before mixing it well. Let the chili boil and then reduce heat to cook it without covering the skillet on low heat for 30 to 45 minutes. Serve with green onion on the top.

Recipe 07: Squash Soup For Dinner

- 3 lbs butternut squash, peeled and chopped
- 1 cup chopped shallots
- 1/2 teaspoon salt
- 1 bay leaf
- 3 cloves garlic, chopped
- 1 cup chicken broth, without salt

- 2 teaspoons olive oil

- 1 cup vegetable broth, without salt

- 14-ounce coconut milk

Ingredients to Garnish:

- Paprika

- Cilantro

- Black pepper powder

- Sunflower seeds

Directions:

Prepare oven at 450° F and add oil and salt on the squash and onion on a baking sheet and then bake for 25 to 30 minutes. You can mix it once or twice. Now add these baked vegetables in a large pan and add remaining oil to cook for 3 to 5 minutes on medium heat. Now cook after adding garlic for 30 seconds. It is time to add milk, broth, and bay leaves and let it simmer for 5 minutes on medium heat. Now discard bay leaves and blend squash mixture in a blender to make a smooth puree.

Chapter 5: 10+ Common Mistakes People Make In Paleo Diet

Nowadays, health conscious people are looking for different ways to remain healthy and stress-free. It is important to return to the caveman diet in which, you can consume natural fruits and vegetables. You have to return to the 40,000 years old diet and reduce farming and industrial food items. Make sure to consume real food grown in a natural environment. The paleo diet is a great way to include natural meals in your diet, but there are some common mistakes that you should avoid:

People Consider it a High Protein Diet

It is not a high protein diet, but you have to include high-quality protein in your diet. The protein and fibers are found in different fruits and vegetables. You have to consume a balanced amount of protein because excessive protein can increase acidity in your body.

It is not a Zero-Carb Diet

You have to avoid high-carb consumption, but this diet is not about completely cutting the consumption of carbohydrates. You can take sweet potatoes and other tubers to include low carb vegetables in your diet. You need intensive training and strategic consumption of carbs.

It is not about all or nothing

There are various versions of Paleo diet and you have to select your own version. There are some simple principles that should be followed on all versions of paleo diet:

- Remove processed foods from the diet
- Remove gluten food
- Avoid vegetable oils
- Get rid of sugars

You should follow these principles to enjoy better health because this diet will help you to feel good.

Avoiding Enough Assortment Carbohydrates

You have to include an assortment of carbohydrates in your diet, the zucchini, green veggies, and Broccoli are good sources of carbs. You can include these vegetables in your diet to get vitamins, enzymes, and minerals. It is good for your body cells and digestive system.

It is not only a weight loss program

Paleo is a good lifestyle in which you have to remove processed and high sugar food items. You will include clean and unprocessed food in your diet to get energy. Keep it in mind that it is not a weight loss program, but the clean eating principles will make you slim.

It is not a Detox Program

Some people think that paleo is a detox program because they remove sugar, processed food, and salt in your diet. This type of diet plan will help you to remove toxins from your body and you can get closer to a healthy life. You will remove all chemicals and additives from your diet.

Starting Without Planning

Lots of people make a mistake by starting paleo diet without planning. You have to plan everything in advance while following a paleo lifestyle. You should have a shopping list and write all ingredients that you want to buy to prepare healthy meals.

Portion Deformation

Some people often move to this life after gaining weight and they follow it step by step. You need to prepare a diet plan with low calories because in order to reduce weight, you should reduce your calorie intake. The nuts, oil, coconut butter like foods are consumed in moderation and you are not allowed to have their high consumption.

Not Become a Discernible Shopper

If a food packet has "gluten-free" label, it doesn't mean that it is healthy. The label may misguide you; therefore, you should read ingredients before buying any diet food.

Holistic Lifestyle with Lots of Health

Paleo diet is referred as a holistic lifestyle with healthy food, but you have to focus on exercises and enough sleep as well. If you want to get good health, then make sure to focus on each and every aspect of this diet. Sufficient sleep is necessary to reduce stress, hormone and regulate metabolism.

Fear for Fat

If you want to get actual benefits of Paleo diet, then it is time to get rid of fat phobias. There are some quality fats, such as olives, coconut oil, olive oil, flaxseeds, and pasture butter, avocado that are good to nourish your brain. These can improve your insulin sensitivity and regulate good hormones. Healthy sugar in your body can help you to reduce cholesterol and fat.

Paleo Diet

Paleo Salmon And Chili Sauce

(Prep + Cook Time: 25 minutes | Servings: 12)

Ingredients:

- 1¼ cups coconut; shredded
- 1 lb. salmon; cut into medium cubes
- 1/3 cup coconut flour
- A pinch of sea salt
- Black pepper to the taste
- 1 egg
- 2 tbsp. coconut oil
- ¼cup water
- 1/4 tsp. agar agar
- 4 red chilies; chopped
- 3 garlic cloves; minced
- 1/4 cup balsamic vinegar
- 1/2 cup honey

Instructions:

1. In a bowl; mix coconut flour with a pinch of salt and stir.
2. In another bowl; whisk the egg with black pepper.
3. Put coconut in a third bowl.
4. Dip salmon cubes in flour, egg and coconut and place them all on a working surface.
5. Heat up a pan with the oil over medium high heat, add salmon cubes, fry them for 3 minutes on each side, transfer them to paper towels, drain grease and divide them between plates.
6. Heat up a pan with the water over medium high heat.
7. Add chilies, cloves, vinegar, honey and agar agar, stir very well, bring to a gentle boil and simmer until all ingredients combine. Drizzle this over salmon cubes and serve.

Nutrition Facts Per Serving: Calories: 140; Fat: 1; Fiber: 2; Carbs: 4; Protein: 15

Paleo Shrimp Dish

(Prep + Cook Time: 20 minutes | Servings: 4)

Ingredients:

- 1 small red bell pepper; chopped
- 1 small yellow onion; chopped
- 20 shrimp; peeled and deveined
- 1 garlic clove; finely chopped
- 5 dried red chilies
- 1 inch ginger; minced
- 1/4 cup coconut aminos
- A pinch of sea salt
- Black pepper to the taste
- 2 tbsp. coconut oil
- 2 tbsp. water
- 1 tbsp. lime juice
- 1 tsp. apple cider vinegar
- 1 tsp. raw honey
- A handful cilantro; finely chopped for serving

Instructions:

1. In a bowl; mix aminos with vinegar, honey, water and lime juice and whisk well.
2. Heat up a pan with the coconut oil over medium heat, add garlic and ginger, stir and cook for 2 minutes.
3. Add red chilies, onion, bell pepper, stir and cook for 4 minutes.
4. Add shrimp, a pinch of salt and pepper to the taste and the vinegar mix you've made, stir and cook for 5 minutes. Divide between plates and serve with cilantro sprinkled on top.

Nutrition Facts Per Serving: Calories: 157; Fat: 7; Carbs: 11; Fiber: 0; Protein: 5

Shrimp And Zucchini Noodles

(Prep + Cook Time: 25 minutes | Servings: 2)

Ingredients:

- 2 zucchinis; sliced in thin noodles
- 1 lb. shrimp; peeled and deveined
- 4 garlic cloves; minced
- A pinch of sea salt
- Black pepper to the taste
- 1/4 cup white wine
- 2 tbsp. chives; chopped
- 2 tbsp. lemon juice
- 2 tbsp. coconut oil

Instructions:

1. Heat up a pan with the coconut oil over medium high heat, add garlic, stir and cook for 3 minutes.
2. Add shrimp, stir and cook for 3 minutes and transfer them to a plate.
3. Pour lemon juice and wine into the pan, bring to a boil over medium heat and simmer for a few minutes.
4. Add zucchini noodles, the shrimp, a pinch of sea salt and pepper to the taste stir gently and divide among plates. Sprinkle chives on top and serve.

Nutrition Facts Per Serving: Calories: 140; Fat: 12; Carbs: 6; Fiber: 3; Protein: 18

Paleo Fish Dish

(Prep + Cook Time: 20 minutes | Servings: 4)

Ingredients:

- 1/4 cup ghee; melted
- 4 halibut fish fillets
- 4 garlic cloves; minced
- 2 tbsp. parsley; chopped

- Zest and juice from 1 lemon
- 1 lemon; sliced
- A pinch of sea salt
- Black pepper to the taste

Instructions:

1. In a bowl; mix garlic with ghee, lemon zest, juice, parsley, a pinch of sea salt and pepper and stir well.
2. Arrange fish in a baking dish, season with pepper to the taste, drizzle the mix you've made, top with lemon slices, introduce in the oven at 425 °F and bake for 15 minutes. Divide between plates and serve warm.

Nutrition Facts Per Serving: Calories: 150; Fat: 19; Carbs: 5; Fiber: 0.4; Protein: 31

Salmon With Avocado Sauce

(Prep + Cook Time: 30 minutes | Servings: 5)

Ingredients:

- 1 tsp. cumin
- 1 tsp. sweet paprika
- 1 tsp. chili powder
- 1 tsp. onion powder
- 1/2 tsp. garlic powder
- 2 lbs. salmon filets; cut into 4 pieces
- A pinch of sea salt
- Black pepper to the taste

For the avocado sauce:

- 2 avocados; pitted, peeled and chopped
- 1 garlic clove; minced
- Juice from 1 lime
- 1 red onion; chopped
- 1 tbsp. extra virgin olive oil
- Black pepper to the taste

- 1 tbsp. cilantro; finely chopped

Instructions:

1. In a bowl; mix paprika with cumin, onion powder, garlic powder, chili powder, a pinch of sea salt and pepper to the taste.
2. Add salmon pieces, toss to coat and keep in the fridge for 20 minutes.
3. Put avocado in a bowl and mash well with a fork.
4. Add red onion, garlic clove, lime juice, olive oil, chopped cilantro and pepper to the taste and stir very well.
5. Take salmon out of the fridge, place it on preheated grill over medium high heat and cook it for 3 minutes.
6. Flip salmon, cook for 3 more minutes and divide on serving plates. Top each salmon piece with avocado sauce and serve.

Nutrition Facts Per Serving: Calories: 150; Fat: 12; Carbs: 9; Fiber: 6; Protein: 24

Glazed Salmon

(Prep + Cook Time: 25 minutes | Servings: 4)

Ingredients:
- 2 tbsp. pure maple syrup
- 4 salmon fillets; skin on
- A pinch of sea salt
- White pepper to the taste
- 2 tsp. Dijon mustard
- Juice and zest from 1 orange
- 2 garlic cloves; finely chopped

Instructions:

1. In a bowl; mix maple syrup with orange zest, juice, mustard, a pinch of sea salt, pepper and garlic and whisk well.

2. Arrange salmon in a baking dish, brush with the maple syrup and orange mix, introduce in the oven at 400 °F and bake for 15 minutes. Divide between plates and serve right away.

Nutrition Facts Per Serving: Calories: 190; Fat: 10; Carbs: 12; Fiber: 0.6; Sugar: 13; Protein: 26

Shrimp And Cauliflower Rice

(Prep + Cook Time: 25 minutes | Servings: 4)

Ingredients:

- 1 tbsp. ghee
- 1 cauliflower head; florets separated
- 1/4 cup coconut milk
- 1 lb. shrimp; peeled and deveined
- 2 garlic cloves; minced
- 8 oz. mushrooms; sliced
- 4 bacon slices
- A pinch of red pepper flakes
- A handful mixed parsley and chives; chopped
- 1/2 cup beef stock
- Black pepper to the taste

Instructions:

1. Heat up a pan over medium high heat, add bacon slices, cook until they are crispy, drain grease on paper towels and leave them aside for now.
2. Put cauliflower florets in your food processor, blend until you obtain your "rice" and transfer to a heated pan over medium high heat.
3. Cook cauliflower rice for 5 minutes stirring often.
4. Add coconut milk and 1 tbsp. ghee, stir and cook for a couple more minutes.

5. Blend everything using an immersion blender, add black pepper to the taste, stir; reduce heat to low and continue cooking for a few minutes more.
6. Heat up the pan where you cooked the bacon over medium high heat, add shrimp, cook for 2 minutes on each side and transfer them to a plate.
7. Heat up the pan again, add mushrooms, stir and cook for a few minutes as well.
8. Add garlic, pepper flakes and some black pepper, stir and cook for 1 minute. Add stock, return shrimp to pan, stir and cook until stock evaporates.
9. Divide cauliflower rice on plates, top with shrimp and mushrooms mix, top with crispy bacon and sprinkle parsley and chives.

Nutrition Facts Per Serving: Calories: 140; Fat: 2; Fiber: 2; Carbs: 4; Protein: 9

Lobster With Sauce

(Prep + Cook Time: 20 minutes | Servings: 4)

Ingredients:
- 1/4 cup ghee; melted
- 4 lobster tails
- A pinch of sea salt
- Black pepper to the taste
- 2 tbsp. Sriracha sauce
- 1 tbsp. lime juice
- 1 tbsp. chives; chopped
- Some parsley leaves; chopped for serving

Instructions:

1. In a bowl; mix Sriracha sauce with ghee, chives, a pinch of sea salt, pepper and lime juice and whisk well.
2. Cut lobster tails halfway through in the center, open with your fingers, fill them with half of the Sriracha mix, arrange

on preheated grill over medium high heat, cook for 4 minutes, flip and cook for 3 minutes more.
3. Divide lobster tails on plates, drizzle the rest of the Sriracha sauce, sprinkle parsley on top and serve.

Nutrition Facts Per Serving: Calories: 240; Fat: 16; Carbs: 2; Fiber: 0.5; Protein: 19

Steamed Clams

(Prep + Cook Time: 20 minutes | Servings: 2)
Ingredients:
- 3 tbsp. ghee
- 1½ lbs. shell clams; scrubbed
- 1/4 cup white wine
- 3 garlic cloves; finely chopped
- A pinch of sea salt
- Black pepper to the taste
- 1/2 cup chicken stock
- 2 tbsp. parsley; chopped
- Lemon wedges

Instructions:
1. Heat up a pot with the ghee over medium heat, add garlic, stir and cook for 1 minute.
2. Add wine, bring to a boil and simmer for a few minutes.
3. Add stock and clams, cover pot and cook for 4-5 minutes.
4. Divide clams on plates, sprinkle parsley on top, a pinch of sea salt and pepper and serve with lemon wedges on the side.

Nutrition Facts Per Serving: Calories: 79; Fat: 23; Carbs: 9; Fiber: 0.4; Protein: 22

Salmon Pie

(Prep + Cook Time: 1 hour 15 minutes | Servings: 4)

Ingredients:

- 8 sweet potatoes; thinly sliced
- 4 cups salmon; already cooked and shredded
- 1 red onion; chopped
- 2 carrots; chopped
- 1 celery stalk; chopped
- A pinch of sea salt
- Black pepper to the taste
- 2 tbsp. chives; chopped
- 2 cups coconut milk
- 1 tbsp. tapioca starch
- 2 garlic cloves; minced
- 3 tbsp. ghee

Instructions:

1. Heat up a pan with the ghee over medium heat, add garlic and tapioca, stir and cook for 1 minute.
2. Add coconut milk, stir and cook for 3 minutes.
3. Add a pinch of sea salt and pepper and stir again.
4. In a bowl; mix carrots with salmon, celery, chives, onion and pepper to the taste and stir well.
5. Arrange a layer of potatoes in a baking dish, add some of the coconut sauce, add half of the salmon mix, the rest of the potatoes and top with the remaining sauce.
6. Introduce in the oven at 375 °F and bake for 1 hour. Divide between plates and serve hot.

Nutrition Facts Per Serving: Calories: 260; Fat: 11; Carbs: 20; Fiber: 12; Protein: 14

Grilled Calamari

(Prep + Cook Time: 15 minutes | Servings: 4)

Ingredients:

- 2 lbs. calamari; tentacles andtubes sliced into rings
- 1 lime; sliced

- 1 lemon; sliced
- 1 orange; sliced
- 2 tbsp. parsley; chopped
- A pinch of sea salt
- Black pepper to the taste
- 3 tbsp. lemon juice
- 1/4 cup extra virgin olive oil
- 2 garlic cloves; minced

Instructions:

1. In a bowl; mix calamari with sliced lemon, lime, orange, lemon juice, a pinch of sea salt, pepper, parsley, garlic and olive oil and toss to coat.
2. Heat up your kitchen grill over medium high heat, add calamari and fruits slices, cook for 5 minutes, divide between plates and serve.

Nutrition Facts Per Serving: Calories: 90; Fat: 3; Carbs: 0.2; Fiber: 0; Protein: 15

Special Paleo Salmon

(Prep + Cook Time: 30 minutes | Servings: 4)

Ingredients:

- 6 cabbage leaves; sliced in half
- 4 medium salmon steaks; skinless
- 2 red bell peppers; chopped
- Some coconut oil
- 1 yellow onion; chopped
- A pinch of sea salt
- Black pepper to the taste

Instructions:

1. Put water in a pot, bring to a boil over medium high heat, add cabbage leaves, blanch them for 2 minutes, transfer to a bowl filled with cold water and pat dry them.
2. Season salmon steaks with a pinch of sea salt and black pepper to the taste and wrap each in 3 cabbage leaf halves.
3. Heat up a pan with some coconut oil over medium high heat, add onion and bell pepper, stir and cook for 4 minutes.
4. Add wrapped salmon, introduce pan in the oven at 350 °F and bake for 12 minutes. Divide salmon and veggies between plates and serve.

Nutrition Facts Per Serving: Calories: 140; Fat: 3; Fiber: 1; Carbs: 2; Protein: 15

Roasted Trout

(Prep + Cook Time: 30 minutes | Servings: 4)

Ingredients:

- 3 trout; cleaned and gutted
- 1 bunch dill
- 2 lemons; sliced
- 1 bunch rosemary
- 2 fennel bulbs; sliced
- A pinch of sea salt
- Black pepper to the taste
- 2 tbsp. extra virgin olive oil

Instructions:

1. Grease a baking dish with some oil, spread fennel slices on the bottom and add trout after you've seasoned them with a pinch of sea salt and pepper.
2. Fill each fish with lemon slices, dill and rosemary springs.
3. Top fish with the rest of the herbs and lemon slices, drizzle the rest of the oil, introduce everything in the oven at 500 °F and bake for 10 minutes.

4. Reduce heat to 425 °F and bake for 12 more minutes. Leave fish to cool down, divide between plates and serve.

Nutrition Facts Per Serving: Calories: 143; Fat: 2.3; Carbs: 1; Fiber: 0; Protein: 6

Roasted Cod

(Prep + Cook Time: 30 minutes | Servings: 4)

Ingredients:
- 1/4 cup ghee
- 4 medium cod fillets; skinless
- 2 garlic cloves; minced
- 1 tbsp. parsley leaves; finely chopped
- 1 tsp. mustard
- 1 shallot; finely chopped
- 3 tbsp. prosciutto; chopped
- 2 tbsp. lemon juice
- 2 tbsp. coconut oil
- A pinch of sea salt
- Black pepper to the taste
- Lemon wedges for serving

Instructions:
1. In a bowl; mix parsley with ghee, mustard, garlic, shallot, prosciutto, a pinch of sea salt, pepper and lemon juice and whisk very well.
2. Heat up an oven proof pan with the coconut oil over medium high heat, add fish, season with black pepper to the taste and cook for 4 minutes on each side.
3. Spread ghee mix over fish, introduce in the oven at 425 °F and bake for 10 minutes. Divide between plates and serve with lemon wedges on the side.

Nutrition Facts Per Serving: Calories: 138; Fat: 4; Carbs: 1; Fiber: 0; Protein: 23

Paleo Salmon Dish

(Prep + Cook Time: 40 minutes | Servings: 6)

Ingredients:

- 2 tbsp. ghee
- A pinch of sea salt
- Black pepper to the taste
- 3 cups apple cider
- 1/2 tsp. fennel seeds
- 1 tsp. mustard seeds
- 1 fennel bulb; chopped
- 1 apple; cored, peeled and chopped
- 4 salmon fillets; skin on and bone in

Instructions:

1. Put cider in a pot and heat up over medium heat.
2. Add mustard seeds, a pinch of salt, black pepper and fennel seeds, stir and boil for 25 minutes.
3. Strain this into a bowl; add half of the ghee, stir well and leave aside for now.
4. Heat up a pan with the rest of the ghee over medium heat, add fennel and apple pieces, stir and cook for 6 minutes.
5. Brush salmon pieces with some of the cider mix, season with a pinch of salt and black pepper, place on a lined baking sheet.
6. Add fennel and apple pieces as well, introduce everything in the oven at 350 °F and bake for 25 minutes. Divide salmon between plates and serve with the rest of the cider sauce on top.

Nutrition Facts Per Serving: Calories: 150; Fat: 3; Fiber: 2; Carbs: 4; Protein: 10

Fish Tacos

(Prep + Cook Time: 25 minutes | Servings: 4)

Ingredients:

- 4 tilapia fillets; cut into medium pieces
- 1/4 cup coconut flour
- 2 eggs
- 3/4 cup tapioca starch
- 1/2 cup tapioca starch
- 1/4 cup sparkling water
- 2 cups cabbage; shredded
- 2 cups coconut oil
- A pinch of sea salt
- Black pepper to the taste
- Lime wedges for serving
- Cauliflower tortillas

For the Pico de Gallo:

- 2 tomatoes; chopped
- 2 tbsp. jalapeno; finely chopped
- 6 tbsp. yellow onion; finely chopped
- 2 tbsp. lime juice
- 1 tbsp. cilantro; finely chopped

For the mayo:

- 1 tbsp. Sriracha sauce
- 1/4 cup homemade mayonnaise
- 2 tsp. lime juice

Instructions:

1. In a bowl; mix tomatoes with tomatoes with onion, jalapeno, cilantro, 2 tbsp. lime juice and stir well, cover and keep in the fridge for now.
2. In another bowl; mix mayo with Sriracha and 2 tsp. lime juice, stir well, cover and also keep in the fridge.
3. In a bowl; mix 3/4 cup tapioca starch with coconut flour, sparkling water, a pinch of sea salt, pepper and eggs and whisk very well.
4. Put the rest of the tapioca starch in a separate bowl.

5. Pat dry tapioca pieces, coat with tapioca starch and dip each piece in eggs mix.
6. Heat up a pan with the coconut oil over medium high heat, transfer fish fillets to pan, cook for 1 minute, flip them, cook for 1 more minute, transfer to paper towels and drain excess fat.
7. Arrange tortillas on a working surface, divide cabbage on them, add a piece of fish on each, add some of the Pico de Gallo and top with mayo. Serve with lime wedges.

Nutrition Facts Per Serving: Calories: 230; Fat: 10; Carbs: 12; Fiber: 4; Protein: 13

It might seem like a very simple dish, but it's a delicious and fresh one!

Paleo Thai Shrimp Delight

(Prep + Cook Time: 60 minutes | Servings: 4)
Ingredients:
- 1 lb. shrimp; peeled and deveined
- 2 shallots; chopped
- 1 spaghetti squash; cut in halves and seedless
- Juice from 1 lime
- 2 tbsp. coconut aminos
- 1 tbsp. chili sauce
- 1 tsp. ginger; grated
- 3 garlic cloves; minced
- 3 cups mung beans sprouts
- 3 tbsp. coconut oil
- 2 tbsp. almond butter
- 2 eggs; whisked
- 1 cup carrots; chopped
- 1/4 cup nuts; roasted and chopped
- 1/4 cup cilantro; chopped

45

- 4 green onions; chopped
- A pinch of sea salt
- Black pepper to the taste

Instructions:

1. Brush squash halves with 1 tbsp. coconut oil, arrange pieces on a lined baking sheet, place in the oven at 400 °F and bake for 40 minutes.
2. Leave squash to cool down and make squash noodles using a fork.
3. Heat up a pan over medium heat, add coconut aminos, lime juice, almond butter and chili sauce and stir well until everything combines.
4. Heat up another pan with the rest of the oil over medium high heat, add shrimp, cook for 4 minutes and transfer to a plate.
5. Heat up the pan again over medium high heat, add ginger, shallots and garlic, stir and cook for 2 minutes.
6. Add carrots and sprouts, stir and cook for 1 minute. Add eggs and stir everything.
7. Add almond butter sauce you've made earlier, squash noodles, cilantro, green onions, nuts, shrimp, a pinch of salt and black pepper, stir well, divide between plates and serve right away.

Nutrition Facts Per Serving: Calories: 150; Fat: 3; Fiber: 2; Carbs: 3; Protein: 14

Paleo Smoked Salmon And Veggies

(Prep + Cook Time: 10 minutes | Servings: 2)

Ingredients:

- 2 cups cherry tomatoes; cut in halves
- 1 red onion; thinly sliced
- 8 oz. smoked salmon; thinly sliced
- 1 cucumber; thinly chopped

- 6 tbsp. extra virgin olive oil
- 1/2 tsp. garlic; minced
- 2 tbsp. lemon juice
- Black pepper to the taste
- 1 tsp. balsamic vinegar
- Some dill; finely chopped
- 1/2 tsp. oregano; dried

Instructions:

1. In a bowl; mix oil with garlic, balsamic vinegar, oregano and garlic and whisk well.
2. Add black pepper to the taste and stir well again.
3. In a bowl; mix cucumber with tomatoes and onion.
4. Drizzle the dressing over veggies and toss to coat.
5. Roll salmon pieces and divide them among plates. Add mixed veggies on the side, sprinkle dill all over and serve.

Nutrition Facts Per Serving: Calories: 159; Fat: 23; Carbs: 2; Fiber: 3; Protein: 14

Paleo Salmon And Lemon Relish

(Prep + Cook Time: 1 hour 10 minutes | Servings: 2)

Ingredients:

- 1 big salmon fillet; cut in halves
- Black pepper to the taste
- A drizzle of olive oil
- A pinch of sea salt

For the relish:

- 1 tbsp. lemon juice
- 1 shallot; chopped
- 1 Meyer lemon; cut in wedges and then thinly sliced
- 2 tbsp. parsley; chopped
- 1/4 cup olive oil
- Black pepper to the taste

Instructions:

1. Put some water in a dish and place it in the oven.
2. Put the salmon on a lined baking dish, drizzle some olive oil, season with a pinch of sea salt and black pepper, rub well, place in the oven at 370 °F and bake for 1 hour.
3. Meanwhile; in a bowl, mix shallot with the lemon juice, a pinch of salt and black pepper, stir and leave aside for 10 minutes.
4. In another bowl; mix marinated shallot with lemon slices, some salt, pepper, parsley and 1/4 cup oil and whisk well. Cut salmon in chunks, divide on plates and top with lemon relish.

Nutrition Facts Per Serving: Calories: 200; Fat: 3; Fiber: 3; Carbs: **6; Protein: 20**

Scallops With Delicious Puree

(Prep + Cook Time: 35 minutes | Servings: 4)

Ingredients:

- 3 garlic cloves; minced
- 2 cups cauliflower florets; chopped
- 2 cups sweet potatoes; chopped
- 2 rosemary springs
- 12 sea scallops
- A pinch of sea salt
- Black pepper to the taste
- 1/4 cup pine nuts; toasted
- 2 cups veggie stock
- 2 tbsp. extra virgin olive oil
- A handful chives; chopped

Instructions:

1. Put cauliflower, potatoes and stock in a pot, bring to a boil over medium high heat, reduce temperature and simmer until veggies are soft.
2. Drain veggies, transfer them to your blender, add a pinch of sea salt and pepper to the taste and pulse until you obtain a puree.
3. Heat up a pan with the oil over medium high heat, add rosemary and garlic, stir and cook for 1 minute.
4. Add scallops, cook them for 2 minutes, often stirring, season them with pepper to the taste and take them off heat. Divide puree on small plates, arrange scallops on top, sprinkle chives and pine nuts at the end and serve.

Nutrition Facts Per Serving: Calories: 170; Fat: 10; Fiber: 0; Carbs: 2; Protein: 22

Paleo Tuna And Chimichurri Sauce

(Prep + Cook Time: 15 minutes | Servings: 4)

Ingredients:

- 1 small red onion; chopped
- 1/2 cup cilantro; chopped
- 1/3 cup olive oil
- 2 tbsp. olive oil
- 1 jalapeno pepper; chopped
- 2 tbsp. basil; chopped
- 3 tbsp. vinegar
- 3 garlic cloves; minced
- 1 tsp. red pepper flakes
- 1 tsp. thyme; chopped
- A pinch of sea salt
- Black pepper to the taste
- 1 lb. sushi grade tuna
- 2 avocados; pitted, peeled and chopped
- 6 oz. arugula

Instructions:

1. In a bowl; mix 1/3 cup oil with onion, jalapeno, cilantro, basil, vinegar, garlic, parsley, pepper flakes, thyme, a pinch of salt and black pepper and whisk well.
2. Heat up a pan with 2 tbsp. oil over medium high heat, add tuna, season with a pinch of sea salt and black pepper, cook for 2 minutes on each side, transfer to a cutting board, leave aside to cool down and slice.
3. In a bowl; mix arugula with half of the chimichurri sauce you've made earlier, toss to coat well and divide between plates. Divide tuna slices, avocado pieces and drizzle the rest of the sauce on top.

Nutrition Facts Per Serving: Calories: 140; Fat: 1; Fiber: 1; Carbs: 2; Protein: 6

Paleo Tuna Dish

(Prep + Cook Time: 25 minutes | Servings: 4)

Ingredients:

- 1 tsp. fennel seeds
- 1 tsp. mustard seeds
- 4 medium tuna steaks
- 1/4 tsp. black peppercorns
- A pinch of sea salt
- Black pepper to the taste
- 4 tbsp. sesame seeds
- 3 tbsp. coconut oil

Instructions:

1. In your grinder, mix peppercorns with fennel and mustard seeds and grind well.
2. Add sesame seeds, a pinch of sea salt and pepper to the taste and grind again well.
3. Spread this mix on a plate, add tuna steaks and toss to coat.

4. Heat up a pan with the oil over medium high heat, add tuna steaks and cook for 3 minutes on each side. Divide between plates and serve with a side salad.

Nutrition Facts Per Serving: Calories: 240; Fat: 2; Carbs: 0; Fiber: 0; Protein: 53

Paleo Salmon Tartar Delight

(Prep + Cook Time: 15 minutes | Servings: 4)

Ingredients:

- 7 oz. smoked salmon; minced
- 14 oz. salmon fillet; cut into very small cubes
- 3 tbsp. red onion; minced
- 2 tbsp. pickled cucumber; minced
- Zest and juice from 1 lemon
- 1 garlic clove; finely minced
- 2 tbsp. basil; minced
- 2 tsp. oregano; dried
- Black pepper to the taste
- 2 tbsp. mint leaves; minced
- 2 tbsp. Dijon mustard
- 5 tbsp. extra virgin olive oil
- Lime wedges for serving

Instructions:

1. In a bowl; mix onion with cucumber, garlic, lemon zest and juice, basil, mint, oregano, mustard, oil and pepper and stir well.
2. Add smoked and fresh salmon and stir well again. Divide tartar between plates and serve with lime wedges on the side.

Nutrition Facts Per Serving: Calories: 230; Fat: 16; Carbs: 2.3; Fiber: 0.4; Protein: 17

Paleo Grilled Salmon With Peaches

(Prep + Cook Time: 25 minutes | Servings: 4)

Ingredients:

- 2 red onions; cut into wedges
- 3 peaches; cut in wedges
- 4 salmon steaks
- 1 tsp. thyme; chopped
- 1 tbsp. ginger; grated
- A pinch of sea salt
- Black pepper to the taste
- 1 tbsp. white wine vinegar
- 3 tbsp. extra virgin olive oil

Instructions:

1. In a bowl; mix wine with ginger, vinegar, thyme, a pinch of sea salt, pepper and olive oil and whisk very well.
2. In a bowl; mix peaches with onion, salt and pepper and toss to coat.
3. Heat up your kitchen grill over medium high heat, add salmon steaks after you've seasoned them with pepper to the taste, grill for 6 minutes on each side and divide between plates.
4. Add peaches and onions to grill, cook for 4 minutes on each side and transfer next to salmon on plates. Drizzle the vinaigrette you've made all over salmon, onions and peaches and serve right away.

Nutrition Facts Per Serving: Calories: 448; Fat: 26; Carbs: 13; Fiber: 2; Sugar: 8; Protein: 40

Shrimp Burgers

(Prep + Cook Time: 30 minutes | Servings: 4)

Ingredients:

- 2 tbsp. cilantro; chopped
- 1½ lbs. shrimp; peeled and deveined
- 2 tbsp. chives; chopped
- Black pepper to the taste
- 1 garlic clove; minced
- 1/4 cup radishes; minced
- 1 tsp. lemon zest
- 1/4 cup celery; minced
- 1 egg; whisked
- 1 tbsp. lemon juice
- 1/4 cup almond meal

For the salsa:

- 1 avocado; pitted, peeled and chopped
- 1 cup pineapple; chopped
- 2 tbsp. red onion; chopped
- 1/4 cup bell peppers; chopped
- 1 tbsp. lime juice
- 1 tbsp. cilantro; finely chopped
- A pinch of sea salt
- Black pepper to the taste

Instructions:

1. In a bowl; mix pineapple with avocado, bell peppers, 2 tbsp. red onion, 1 tbsp. lime juice, pepper to the taste and 1 tbsp. cilantro, stir well and keep in the fridge for now.
2. In your food processor, mix shrimp with 2 tbsp. cilantro, chives and garlic and blend well.
3. Transfer to a bowl and mix with radishes, celery, lemon zest, lemon juice, egg, almond meal, a pinch of sea salt and pepper to the taste and stir well.
4. Shape 4 burgers, place them on preheated grill over medium high heat and cook for 5 minutes on each side. Divide shrimp burgers between plates and serve with the salsa you've made earlier on the side.

Nutrition Facts Per Serving: Calories: 238; Fat: 12; Carbs: 13.2; Fiber: 3; Protein: 15.4

Scallops Tartar

(Prep + Cook Time: 15 minutes | Servings: 2)

Ingredients:

- 6 scallops; diced
- A pinch of sea salt
- Black pepper to the taste
- 3 strawberries; chopped
- 1 tbsp. extra virgin olive oil
- 1 tbsp. green onions; minced
- Juice from 1/2 lemon
- 1/2 tbsp. basil leaves; finely chopped

Instructions:

1. In a bowl; mix strawberries with scallops, basil and onions and stir well.
2. Add olive oil, a pinch of salt, pepper to the taste and lemon juice and stir well again. Keep in the fridge until you serve.

Nutrition Facts Per Serving: Calories: 180; Fat: 27; Carbs: 3; Fiber: 0; Protein: 24

Salmon And Spicy Slaw

(Prep + Cook Time: 16 minutes | Servings: 4)

Ingredients:

- 3 cups cold water
- 3 scallions; chopped
- 2 tsp. sriracha sauce
- 4 tsp. honey
- 3 tsp. avocado oil
- 4 tsp. cider vinegar
- 2 tsp. flax seed oil

- 4 medium salmon fillets; skinless and boneless
- A pinch of sea salt
- 1½ tsp. jerk seasoning
- 2 cups cabbage; chopped
- 4 cups baby arugula
- 2 cups radish; julienne cut
- 1/4 cup pepitas; toasted

Instructions:

1. Put scallions in a bowl; add cold water to them and leave aside.
2. In a bowl; mix Sriracha with honey and stir well.
3. In another bowl; combine 2 tsp. of the honey mix with 2 tsp. avocado oil, vinegar, a pinch of sea salt and black pepper and stir well.
4. Sprinkle salmon fillets with a pinch of sea salt, black pepper and jerk seasoning and rub well.
5. Heat up a pan with the rest of the avocado oil over medium high heat, add salmon, cook for 6 minutes, flip, take off heat, cover pan and leave aside for a few more minutes.
6. In a salad bowl; mix cabbage with arugula, radish, pepitas, a pinch of salt, black pepper, the honey and vinegar salad dressing and flax seed oil and toss to coat well.
7. Divide salmon on plates, drizzle the rest of the Sriracha sauce, add cabbage salad next to them and top with drained scallions.

Nutrition Facts Per Serving: Calories: 180; Fat: 3; Fiber: 3; Carbs: 4; Protein: 8

Shrimp Skewers

(Prep + Cook Time: 20 minutes | Servings: 4)

Ingredients:

- 1/2 lb. sausages; chopped and already cooked
- 1/2 lb. shrimp; peeled and deveined

- 2 tbsp. extra virgin olive oil
- 2 zucchinis; cubed
- A pinch of sea salt
- Black pepper to the taste

For the Creole seasoning:
- 1/2 tbsp. garlic powder
- 2 tbsp. paprika
- 1/2 tbsp. onion powder
- 1/4 tbsp. oregano; dried
- 1/2 tbsp. chili powder
- 1/4 tbsp. thyme; dried

Instructions:

1. In a bowl; mix paprika with garlic powder, onion one, chili powder, oregano and thyme and stir well.
2. In another bowl; mix shrimp with sausage, zucchini and oil and toss to coat.
3. Pour paprika mix over shrimp mix and stir well.
4. Arrange sausage, shrimp and zucchini on skewers alternating pieces, season with a pinch of sea salt and black pepper, place them on preheated grill over medium high heat and cook for 8 minutes, flipping skewers from time to time. Arrange on a platter and serve.

Nutrition Facts Per Serving: Calories: 360; Fat: 32; Carbs: 4.3; Fiber: 0.8; Sugar: 1; Protein: 18.1

Paleo Salmon Skewers

(Prep + Cook Time: 25 minutes | Servings: 4)

Ingredients:
- 1 lb. wild salmon; skinless, boneless and cubed
- 2 Meyer lemons; sliced
- 1/4 cup balsamic vinegar
- 1/4 cup orange juice

- 1/3 cup Paleo orange marmalade
- A pinch of pink salt
- Black pepper to the taste

Instructions:

1. Heat up a small pot with the vinegar over medium heat, add marmalade and orange juice, stir; bring to a simmer for 1 minute and take off heat.
2. Skewer salmon cubes and lemon slices, season with a pinch of salt and black pepper, brush them with half of the vinegar mix, place on preheated grill over medium heat, cook for 4 minutes on each side.
3. Brush skewers with the rest of the vinegar mix, grill for 1 minute more, divide between plates and serve.

Nutrition Facts Per Serving: Calories: 150; Fat: 1; Fiber: 2; Carbs: 4; Protein: 10

Paleo Glazed Salmon

(Prep + Cook Time: 50 minutes | Servings: 2)

Ingredients:

- 1 big salmon fillet; cut in halves
- 2 tbsp. mustard
- 1 tbsp. maple syrup
- A pinch of sea salt
- Black pepper to the taste
- 2 sweet potatoes; peeled and chopped
- 2 tsp. coconut oil
- 1/4 cup coconut milk
- 3 garlic cloves; minced

Instructions:

1. In a bowl; mix maple syrup with mustard and whisk well.
2. Season salmon halves with a pinch of sea salt and black pepper to the taste and brush them with half of the maple mix.

3. Heat up a pan with 1 tsp. coconut oil over medium high heat, add salmon, skin side down and cook for 4 minutes.
4. Transfer salmon to a baking dish, brush with the rest of the maple syrup mix, place in the oven at 425 °F and roast for 10 minutes.
5. Put sweet potatoes in a pot, add water to cover, bring to a boil over medium heat, cover and cook for 20 minutes.
6. Heat up a pan with the rest of the oil over medium heat, add garlic, stir and cook for 1 minute.
7. Add sweet potatoes, stir well and then mash everything with a potato masher.
8. Add coconut milk, a pinch of salt and black pepper to the taste and blend using an immersion blender. Divide this mash between plates, add salmon on the side and serve.

Nutrition Facts Per Serving: Calories: 200; Fat: 3; Fiber: 3; Carbs: 6; Protein: 20

Paleo Infused Clams

(Prep + Cook Time: 22 minutes | Servings: 2)

Ingredients:
- 1 tbsp. olive oil
- 3 oz. pancetta
- 3 tbsp. ghee
- 2 lb. little clams; scrubbed
- 1 shallot; minced
- 2 garlic cloves; minced
- 1 bottle infused cider
- 1 apple; cored and chopped
- Juice of 1/2 lemon

Instructions:

1. Heat up a pan with the oil over medium high heat, add pancetta and brown for 3 minutes.
2. Add ghee, shallot and garlic, stir and cook for 3 minutes.

3. Add cider, stir well and cook for 1 minute.
4. Add clams and thyme, cover and simmer for 5 minutes. Add apple and lemon juice, stir; divide everything into bowls and serve.

Nutrition Facts Per Serving: Calories: 120; Fat: 1; Fiber: 2; Carbs: 4; Protein: 10

Paleo Shrimp Dish

(Prep + Cook Time: 15 minutes | Servings: 4)

Ingredients:

- 1 lb. big shrimp; peeled and deveined
- 2 tsp. olive oil
- 1 cup cilantro; chopped
- 1 cup parsley; chopped
- Juice from 2 limes
- 1/2 cup olive oil
- 1/4 cup onion; chopped
- A pinch of sea salt
- 1/2 tsp. smoked paprika
- 2 garlic cloves; minced

Instructions:

1. Heat up a pan with 2 tsp. olive oil over medium heat, add shrimp, cook them for 5 minutes and reduce heat to low.
2. In your food processor, mix 1/2 cup oil with onion, sea salt, paprika, garlic, lime juice, parsley and cilantro and pulse really well. Divide shrimp on plates, top with the chimichurri and serve.

Nutrition Facts Per Serving: Calories: 120; Fat: 2; Fiber: 1; Carbs: 3; Protein: 8

Crab Cakes And Red Pepper Sauce

(Prep + Cook Time: 17 minutes | Servings: 8)

Ingredients:

- 1 cup crab meat
- 2 tbsp. parsley; chopped
- 2 tbsp. old bay seasoning
- 2 tsp. Dijon mustard
- 1 egg; whisked
- 1 tbsp. lemon juice
- 2 tbsp. coconut oil
- 1½ tbsp. coconut flour

For the sauce:

- 1 tbsp. olive oil
- 1/4 cup roasted red peppers
- 1 tbsp. lemon juice
- 1/4 cup avocado; peeled and chopped

Instructions:

1. In a bowl; mix crabmeat with old bay seasoning, parsley, mustard, egg, 1 tbsp. lemon juice and coconut flour and stir everything very well.
2. Shape 8 patties from this mix and place them on a plate.
3. Heat up a pan with 2 tbsp. coconut oil over medium high heat, add crab patties, cook for 3 minutes on each side and divide between plates.
4. In your food processor, mix olive oil with red peppers, avocado and 1 tbsp. lemon juice and blend really well. Spread this on your crab patties and serve.

Nutrition Facts Per Serving: Calories: 100; Fat: 4; Fiber: 3; Carbs: 5; Protein: 7

Grilled Oysters

(Prep + Cook Time: 17 minutes | Servings: 7)

Ingredients:

- 1/4 cup red onion; chopped
- 2 tomatoes; chopped
- A handful cilantro; chopped
- 1 jalapeno; chopped
- A pinch of sea salt
- Black pepper to the taste
- Juice from 1 lime
- 2 limes; cut into wedges
- 24 oysters; scrubbed

Instructions:

1. In a bowl; tomatoes with onion, cilantro, jalapeno, a pinch of salt, black pepper and juice from 1 lime, stir well and leave aside.
2. Heat up your grill over medium high heat, add oysters, grill them for 7 minutes.
3. Open them completely and divide oysters between plates. Top with the tomatoes mix and serve with lime wedges on the side.

Nutrition Facts Per Serving: Calories: 140; Fat: 2; Fiber: 2; Carbs: 4; Protein: 8

Squid And Guacamole

(Prep + Cook Time: 15 minutes | Servings: 2)

Ingredients:

- 2 medium squid; cleaned, tentacles and tubes separated
- A pinch of sea salt
- Black pepper to the taste
- 1 tbsp. olive oil
- Juice of 1/2 lime

For the guacamole:
- 1 tbsp. coriander; chopped
- 2 red chilies; chopped
- 2 avocados; pitted, peeled and chopped
- 1 tomato; chopped
- 1 red onion; chopped
- Juice from 2 limes

Instructions:

1. In a bowl; mix chilies with avocados, coriander, tomato, red onion and juice from 2 limes and stir well.
2. Heat up your grill over medium high heat, add squid pieces after you've rubbed it with 1 tbsp. olive oil, season with salt and pepper to the taste, grill for 3 minutes, flip and cook for 2 minutes on the other side.
3. Transfer squid to a cutting board, slice, drizzle juice from 1/2 lime toss to coat and divide between plates. Serve with the guacamole on the side.

Nutrition Facts Per Serving: Calories: 360; Fat: 7; Fiber: 5; Carbs: 8; Protein: 17

Tasty Stuffed Calamari

(Prep + Cook Time: 1 hour 5 minutes | Servings: 4)

Ingredients:
- 4 big calamari; tentacles separated and chopped
- 2 tbsp. parsley; chopped
- 5 oz. kale; chopped
- 2 garlic cloves; minced
- 1 red bell pepper; chopped
- 1 tsp. oregano; dried
- 14 oz. canned tomato puree
- Some bacon fat
- 1 onion; chopped
- A pinch of sea salt

- Black pepper to the taste

Instructions:

1. Heat up a pan with some bacon fat over medium heat, add onion and garlic, stir and cook for 2 minutes.
2. Add bell pepper, stir and cook for 3 minutes.
3. Add calamari tentacles, stir and cook for 6 minutes more.
4. Add kale, a pinch of sea salt and black pepper, stir; cook for a couple more minutes and take off heat.
5. Stuff calamari tubes with this mix and secure with toothpicks.
6. Heat up a pan with some bacon fat over medium high heat, add calamari, brown them for 2 minutes on each side and then mix with tomato puree.
7. Also add parsley, oregano and some black pepper to the pan, stir gently, cover, reduce heat to medium-low and simmer for 40 minutes. Divide stuffed calamari on plates and serve.

Nutrition Facts Per Serving: Calories: 222; Fat: 10; Fiber: 1; Carbs: 7; Protein: 15

Paleo Tilapia Surprise

(Prep + Cook Time: 35 minutes | Servings: 4)

Ingredients:
- 28 oz. canned coconut milk
- 2 red bell peppers; seedless and cut in halves
- 4 tilapia fillets
- 2 green onions; chopped
- 4 tbsp. Thai red curry paste
- A drizzle of olive oil
- 1/2 cup water
- 2 tbsp. coconut aminos
- 8 lime wedges
- 1 cup basil; chopped

- A pinch of sea salt
- Black pepper to the taste

Instructions:

1. In your food processor, mix half of the coconut milk with basil, curry paste and blend well.
2. Heat up a pan over medium heat, add curry mix and cook for 3 minutes.
3. Add the rest of the coconut milk, water and coconut aminos, stir and cook for 10 minutes.
4. In a bowl; mix fish with bell pepper, a drizzle of oil, a pinch of salt and black pepper to the taste.
5. Heat up a grill over medium high heat, add peppers, grill them for 5 minutes and transfer to a plate.
6. Place fish on the grill, cook for 6 minutes and divide between plates. Add bell peppers on the side, sprinkle green onions, drizzle curry sauce and serve with lime wedges on the side.

Nutrition Facts Per Serving: Calories: 160; Fat: 3; Fiber: 1; Carbs: 2; Protein: 12

Paleo Stuffed Salmon Fillets

(Prep + Cook Time: 30 minutes | Servings: 2)

Ingredients:

- 2 medium salmon fillets; boneless
- 5 oz. tiger shrimp; peeled, deveined and chopped
- 6 mushrooms; chopped
- 3 green onions; chopped
- 2 cups spinach; chopped
- 1/4 cup macadamia nuts; toasted and chopped
- A pinch of sea salt
- Black pepper to the taste
- A pinch of nutmeg; ground
- 1/4 cup Paleo mayonnaise
- Bacon fat for cooking

Instructions:

1. Heat up a pan with some bacon fat over medium heat, add onions and mushrooms, a pinch of salt and black pepper, stir and cook for 4 minutes.
2. Add nuts, stir and cook for 2 minutes more.
3. Add spinach, stir and cook for 1 minute.
4. Add shrimp, stir and cook for another minute.
5. Take this mix off heat, leave it aside to cool down a bit, add Paleo mayo and nutmeg and stir everything.
6. Make an incision lengthwise in each salmon fillet, season with some black pepper and stuff with the shrimp mix.
7. Heat up a pan with some bacon fat over high heat, add salmon fillets and cook skin side down for 1 minute.
8. Cover the pan, reduce temperature to medium-low and cook for 8 minutes more.
9. Introduce pan in preheated broiler and broil for 2 minutes. Divide stuffed salmon fillets on plates and serve.

Nutrition Facts Per Serving: Calories: 450; Fat: 6; Fiber: 4; Carbs: 7; Protein: 40

Paleo Crusted Salmon

(Prep + Cook Time: 30 minutes | Servings: 4)

Ingredients:

- 1 cup pistachios; chopped
- 4 salmon fillets
- 1/4 cup lemon juice
- 2 tbsp. honey
- 1 tsp. dill; chopped
- A pinch of sea salt
- Black pepper to the taste
- 1 tbsp. mustard

Instructions:

1. In a bowl; mix pistachios with mustard, honey, lemon juice, a pinch of salt, black pepper and dill and stir well.
2. Spread this over salmon fillets, press well, place them on a lined baking sheet, place in the oven at 375 °F and bake for 20 minutes. Divide salmon between plates and serve with a side salad.

Nutrition Facts Per Serving: Calories: 150; Fat: 3; Fiber: 2; Carbs: 5; Protein: 12

Paleo Cod And Herb Sauce

(Prep + Cook Time: 25 minutes | Servings: 4)

Ingredients:
- 1 tbsp. chives; chopped
- 4 medium cod fillets
- 1 tbsp. thyme; chopped
- 1 tbsp. parsley; chopped
- Grated zest from 1/2 lemon
- 1 shallot; chopped
- 3/4 cup coconut milk
- 6 tbsp. ghee
- 2 garlic cloves
- A pinch of sea salt
- Black pepper to the taste

Instructions:
1. In a bowl; mix garlic with ghee, shallots, chives, parsley and thyme and stir well.
2. Season cod with a pinch of salt and black pepper to the taste.
3. Heat up a pan over medium heat, add herbed ghee and fish, toss to coat and cook for 2 minutes on each side.
4. Transfer fish to a lined baking sheet, place in the oven at 400 °F and bake for 7 minutes.

5. Heat up the pan with the herbed ghee over medium heat, add lemon zest and coconut milk, stir and bring to a simmer over medium heat. Divide fish on plates, drizzle the herbed sauce on top and serve.

Nutrition Facts Per Serving: Calories: 160; Fat: 3; Fiber: 2; Carbs: 3; Protein: 14

Tasty Spicy Shrimp

(Prep + Cook Time: 14 minutes | Servings: 2)

Ingredients:
- 12 jumbo shrimp; peeled and deveined
- A pinch of sea salt
- Black pepper to the taste
- 2 garlic cloves; minced
- 2 tbsp. olive oil
- 1/4 tsp. red pepper flakes
- 1 tsp. steak seasoning
- 1 tsp. lemon zest
- 1 tbsp. parsley; chopped
- 2 tsp. lemon juice

Instructions:
1. Heat up a pan with the oil over medium high heat, add pepper flakes, garlic and shrimp, stir and cook for 4 minutes.
2. Season with a pinch of sea salt, black pepper, parsley, lemon juice and lemon zest, stir well, divide between plates and serve.

Nutrition Facts Per Serving: Calories: 152; Fat: 12; Fiber: 1; Carbs: 2; Protein: 6

Paleo Mussels Mix

(Prep + Cook Time: 25 minutes | Servings: 6)

Ingredients:
- 3 garlic cloves; minced
- 1 yellow onion; chopped
- 1 tbsp. olive oil
- 1 handful parsley; chopped
- 1/2 cup white wine
- 1 tsp. red pepper flakes
- 28 oz. canned tomatoes; chopped
- 2 cups chicken stock
- 29 oz. canned crushed tomatoes
- 2 lbs. mussels; scrubbed

Instructions:
1. Heat up a pot with the oil over medium heat, add onions, garlic, parsley and pepper flakes, stir and cook for 2 minutes.
2. Add wine, crushed and chopped tomatoes, black pepper and stock, stir; cover and bring to a boil.
3. Add mussels, stir; cover and cook until they open. Ladle this into bowls and serve.

Nutrition Facts Per Serving: Calories: 150; Fat: 3; Fiber: 2; Carbs: 6; Protein: 12

Paleo Mahi Mahi Dish

(Prep + Cook Time: 20 minutes | Servings: 4)

Ingredients:
- 1
- tbsp. chili powder 4 mahi-mahi fillets
- 1/2 tbsp. sweet paprika
- 1/2 tsp. garlic powder
- 1/2 tsp. oregano; dried
-
- 2 tbsp. olive oil
- 2 tbsp. coconut oil

- 1/2 tsp. onion powder
- A handful cilantro; chopped
- Lime wedges

For the cilantro butter:
- Juice of 1 lemon
- 1 garlic clove; minced
- 1/4 cup ghee; melted
- 2 tbsp. cilantro; chopped

Instructions:

1. In a bowl; mix 1/4 cup ghee with 1 garlic clove, juice from 1 lemon and 2 tbsp. cilantro, whisk very well and leave aside for now.
2. In another bowl; mix garlic powder with onion powder, chili powder, oregano and paprika and stir well.
3. Season mahi-mahi with this mix, drizzle the olive oil over them and rub well.
4. Heat up a pan with the coconut oil over medium high heat, add fish fillets, cook for 4 minutes on each side and divide them between plates. Add cilantro butter over fish and serve.

Nutrition Facts Per Serving: Calories: 160; Fat: 4; Fiber: 3; Carbs: 6; Protein: 15

Paleo Halibut And Tasty Salsa

(Prep + Cook Time: 25 minutes | Servings: 4)

Ingredients:
- 4 medium halibut fillets
- 2 tsp. olive oil
- 4 tsp. lemon juice
- 1 garlic clove; minced
- 1 tsp. sweet paprika
- A pinch of sea salt
- Black pepper to the taste

For the salsa:
- 1/4 cup green onions; chopped
- 1 cup red bell pepper; chopped
- 4 tsp. oregano; chopped
- 1 small habanero pepper; chopped
- 1 garlic clove; minced
- 1/4 cup lemon juice

Instructions:

1. In a bowl; mix red bell pepper with habanero, green onion, 1/4 cup lemon juice, 1 garlic clove, oregano, a pinch of sea salt and black pepper, stir well and keep in the fridge for now.
2. In a large bowl; mix paprika, olive oil, 1 garlic clove and 4 tsp. lemon juice and stir well.
3. Add fish, rub well, cover bowl and leave aside for 10 minutes.
4. Place marinated fish on preheated grill over medium high heat, season with a pinch of sea salt and black pepper, cook for 4 minutes on each side and divide between plates. Top fish with the salsa you've made earlier and serve.

Nutrition Facts Per Serving: Calories: 150; Fat: 3; Fiber: 2; Carbs: 3; Protein: 12

Lobster And Sauce

(Prep + Cook Time: 18 minutes | Servings: 4)

Ingredients:
- 2 tbsp.
- ; chopped
- 1 tbsp. parsley; chopped
- 1 tbsp. lime sriracha sauce
- 4 lobster tails; cut halfway through the center
- 1/4 cup ghee; melted

- 1 tbsp. chives juice
- A pinch of sea salt
- Black
1. ; mix ghee with a pinch of salt, black pepper, lime juice, chives and sriracha sauce and whisk well.
- Fill pepper to the taste

Instructions:

2. In a bowl lobster tails with half of this mix, place them on heated grill over medium high heat, cook for 5 minutes, flip, grill them for 3 minutes more and divide between plates.
3. Top lobster tails with the rest of the Sriracha sauce and parsley.

Nutrition Facts Per Serving: Calories: 223; Fat: 12; Fiber: 0; Carbs: 2; Protein: 6

Paleo Grilled Salmon And Avocado Sauce

(Prep + Cook Time: 25 minutes | Servings: 4)

Ingredients:
- 1 avocado; pitted, peeled and chopped
- 4 salmon fillets
- 1/4 cup cilantro; chopped
- 1/3 cup coconut milk
- 1 tbsp. lime juice
- 1 tbsp. lime zest
- 1 tsp. onion powder
- 1 tsp. garlic powder
- A pinch of sea salt
- Black pepper to the taste

Instructions:

1. Season salmon fillets with a pinch of salt, black pepper and lime zest, rub well, place on heated grill over medium heat, cook for 15 minutes flipping once and divide between plates.

2. In your food processor, mix avocado with cilantro, garlic powder, onion powder, lime juice and coconut milk and blend well.
3. Add a pinch of sea salt and some black pepper, blend again and drizzle this over salmon fillets. Serve right away.

Nutrition Facts Per Serving: Calories: 170; Fat: 7; Fiber: 2; Carbs: 3; Protein: 20

Paleo Roasted Cod

(Prep + Cook Time: 30 minutes | Servings: 4)

Ingredients:
- 1 tbsp. parsley; chopped
- 4 medium cod filets
- 1/4 cup ghee
- 2 garlic cloves; minced
- 2 tbsp. bacon fat
- 2 tbsp. lemon juice
- 3 tbsp. prosciutto; chopped
- 1 tsp. Dijon mustard
- 1 shallot; chopped
- A pinch of sea salt
- Black pepper to the taste
- Lemon wedges

Instructions:
1. In a bowl; mix mustard with ghee, garlic, parsley, shallot, lemon juice, prosciutto, salt and pepper and whisk well.
2. Heat up a pan with the bacon fat over medium high heat, add fish fillets, season them with some black pepper and cook for 4 minutes on each side.
3. Spread mustard and ghee mix over fish, transfer everything to a lined baking sheet, place in the oven at 425 °F and bake

for 10 minutes. Divide fish between plates and serve with lemon wedges on the side.

Nutrition Facts Per Serving: Calories: 150; Fat: 4; Fiber: 1; Carbs: 3; Protein: 20

Paleo Grilled Calamari

(Prep + Cook Time: 15 minutes | Servings: 4)

Ingredients:

- 2 lbs. calamari tentacles and tubes cut into rings
- 2 tbsp. parsley; minced
- 1 lemon; sliced
- 1 lime; sliced
- 2 garlic cloves; minced
- 3 tbsp. lemon juice
- 1/4 cup olive oil
- A pinch of sea salt
- Black pepper to the taste

Instructions:

1. In a bowl; mix calamari with parsley, lime slices, lemon slices, garlic, lemon juice, a pinch of salt, black pepper and olive oil and stir well.
2. Place calamari rings on preheated grill over medium high heat, cook for 5 minutes and divide between plates. Serve with the lemon and lime slices and some of the marinade drizzled on top.

Nutrition Facts Per Serving: Calories: 130; Fat: 4; Fiber: 1; Carbs: 3; Protein: 12

Paleo Shrimp With Mango And Avocado Mix

(Prep + Cook Time: 15 minutes | Servings: 2)

Ingredients:

- 1 avocado; pitted, peeled and chopped
- 1 lb. shrimp; peeled and deveined
- 1 tomato; chopped
- 1 mango; peeled and chopped
- 1 jalapeno; chopped
- 1 tbsp. lime juice
- Bacon fat
- 1/4 cup green onions; chopped
- 4 garlic cloves; minced
- A pinch of sea salt
- Black pepper to the taste

Instructions:

1. In a bowl; mix lime juice with jalapeno, mango, tomato, avocado and green onions, stir well and leave aside.
2. Heat up a pan with some bacon fat over medium high heat, add garlic, stir and cook for 2 minutes.
3. Add shrimp, a pinch of sea salt and black pepper, stir and cook for 5 minutes. Divide shrimp on plates, add mango and avocado mix on the side.

Nutrition Facts Per Serving: Calories: 140; Fat: 2; Fiber: 3; Carbs: 3; Protein: 8

Paleo Shrimp And Zucchini Noodles

(Prep + Cook Time: 25 minutes | Servings: 2)

Ingredients:

- 2 zucchinis; cut with a spiralizer
- 1 lb. shrimp; peeled and deveined
- 4 garlic cloves; minced
- 2 tbsp. bacon fat
- 2 tbsp. lemon juice
- 2 tbsp. chives; minced

- A pinch of sea salt
- Black pepper to the taste

Instructions:

1. Heat up a pan with the bacon fat over medium heat, add garlic, stir and cook for 3 minutes.
2. Add shrimp, stir; cook for 4 minutes more and transfer to a plate.
3. Heat up the pan again, add lemon juice and zucchini noodles, stir and cook for 4 minutes.
4. Return shrimp to pan, season with a pinch of salt, black pepper and chives, stir; cook for a couple more minutes and divide between plates. Serve right away.

Nutrition Facts Per Serving: Calories: 140; Fat: 3; Fiber: 3; Carbs: 4; Protein: 8

Paleo Salmon Tartar

(Prep + Cook Time: 30 minutes | Servings: 4)

Ingredients:

- 1 tbsp. chives; minced
- 1 lb. salmon fillet; skinless, boneless and cut into small cubes
- 1 small red onion; chopped
- 1 tbsp. basil; chopped
- Juice fromlemon
- 2 tbsp. capers
- 1/4 cup olive oil
- 1 tsp. mustard
- 2 green onions; chopped
- A pinch of sea salt
- Black pepper to the taste

Instructions:

1. In a big bowl mix chives with onion, basil, capers, salmon and green onions and stir.

2. In another bowl; mix lemon juice with mustard, oil, a pinch of salt and black pepper the taste and stir well. Add this dressing over salad, toss to coat well, divide between plates and serve.

Nutrition Facts Per Serving: Calories: 130; Fat: 1; Fiber: 2; Carbs: 2; Protein: 7

Paleo Salmon Delight

(Prep + Cook Time: 37 minutes | Servings: 4)

Ingredients:
- 10 oz. spinach; chopped
- 5 sun-dried tomatoes; chopped
- 1/4 tsp. red pepper flakes
- 4 medium salmon fillets
- A pinch of sea salt
- Black pepper to the taste
- 1 tbsp. coconut oil
- 1/4 cup shallots; chopped
- 4 garlic cloves

Instructions:
1. Heat up a pan with the oil over medium high heat, add shallots, stir and cook for 3 minutes.
2. Add garlic, stir and cook for 1 minute. Add tomatoes, pepper flakes and spinach, stir and cook for 3 minutes.
3. Season with a pinch of salt and black pepper to the taste, stir; take off heat and leave aside for now.
4. Arrange salmon fillets on a lined baking sheet, season with a pinch of salt and some black pepper, top with the spinach mix, place in the oven at 350 °F and bake for 20 minutes.
5. Divide between plates and serve right away.

Nutrition Facts Per Serving: Calories: 140; Fat: 2; Fiber: 2; Carbs: 3; Protein: 10

Salmon And Chives

(Prep + Cook Time: 22 minutes | Servings: 4)

Ingredients:

- 2 tbsp. dill; chopped
- 4 salmon fillets
- 2 tbsp. chives; chopped
- 1/3 cup maple syrup
- Bacon fat
- 3 tbsp. balsamic vinegar
- A pinch of sea salt
- Black pepper to the taste
- Lime wedges for serving

Instructions:

1. Heat up a pan with bacon fat over medium high heat, add fish fillets, season them with a pinch of sea salt and black pepper, cook for 3 minutes, cover pan and cook for 6 minutes more.
2. Add balsamic vinegar and maple syrup and cook for 3 minutes basting fish with this mix. Add dill and chives, cook for 1 minute, divide fillets between plates and serve with lime wedges on the side.

Nutrition Facts Per Serving: Calories: 140; Fat: 3; Fiber: 2; Carbs: 5; Protein: 10

Paleo Swordfish

(Prep + Cook Time: 16 minutes | Servings: 2)

Ingredients:

- 2 medium wild swordfish fillets
- 1 tbsp. cilantro; chopped
- 1 avocado; pitted, peeled and chopped
- 1 mango; peeled and chopped

- 2 tsp. avocado oil
- 1 tsp. cumin powder
- 1 tsp. onion powder
- 1 tsp. garlic powder
- A pinch of sea salt
- Black pepper to the taste
- 1/2 cup balsamic vinegar
- Juice of 1/2 lime

Instructions:

1. Season fish fillets with a pinch of sea salt, black pepper, onion powder, garlic powder and cumin powder and rub well.
2. Heat up a pan with half of the oil over medium high heat, add fish and vinegar, cook for 3 minutes on each side and transfer to plates.
3. In a bowl; mix avocado with mango, lime juice, cilantro and the rest of the oil and stir well. Divide this salsa next to fish fillets and serve.

Nutrition Facts Per Serving: Calories: 120; Fat: 2; Fiber: 2; Carbs: 4; Protein: 16

Paleo Tuna And Salsa

(Prep + Cook Time: 2 hours 18 minutes | Servings: 4)

Ingredients:

- 1/2 tsp. coriander
- 4 tuna pieces
- A pinch of sea salt
- Black pepper to the taste
- 3 cherry tomatoes; cut in quarters
- 1 red onion; chopped
- 2 avocados; pitted, peeled and chopped
- 2 tbsp. cilantro; chopped

- 2 tbsp. lime juice
- 1 jalapeno; chopped

Instructions:

1. In a bowl; mix cherry tomatoes with avocados, cilantro, lime juice, jalapeno, a pinch of sea salt and black pepper, stir well and keep in the fridge for 2 hours.
2. Season tuna with a pinch of sea salt, black pepper and coriander and rub well.
3. Place tune on preheated grill over medium high heat, cook for 3 minutes on each side and divide between plates. Serve with the avocado salsa on the side.

Nutrition Facts Per Serving: Calories: 150; Fat: 2; Fiber: 1; Carbs: 2; Protein: 14

Paleo Shrimp Cocktail

(Prep + Cook Time: 36 minutes | Servings: 4)

Ingredients:

- 20 jumbo shrimp; deveined but shelled
- 2 cups ice
- A pinch of sea salt
- A drizzle of olive oil
- 1 cup water

For the cocktail sauce:

- 1 cup tomato sauce
- 1/4 tsp. Worcestershire sauce
- Juice of 1 lemon
- Zest from 1 lemon
- 1 tbsp. prepared horseradish
- Chili sauce to the taste

Instructions:

1. In a bowl; mix water with ice, a pinch of sea salt and shrimp, stir; cover and keep in the fridge for 30 minutes.

2. Discard water from shrimp, rinse them, pat dry them, drizzle olive oil over them and rub well.
3. Arrange shrimp on a lined baking sheet, place in preheated broiler and broil them for 3 minutes.
4. Flip, broil for 2 minutes more and leave aside.
5. In a bowl; mix tomato sauce with Worcestershire sauce, lemon juice, lemon zest, chili sauce to the taste and horseradish and whisk well. Arrange shrimp on a platter and serve with the cocktail sauce on the side.

Nutrition Facts Per Serving: Calories: 160; Fat: 3; Fiber: 2; Carbs: 3; Protein: 14

Paleo Crusted Snapper

(Prep + Cook Time: 18 minutes | Servings: 1)
Ingredients:
- 1 red snapper fillet; skinless
- A pinch of sea salt
- Black pepper to the taste
- 1 tbsp. sesame seeds
- 1 tsp. coconut oil

Instructions:

1. Season red snapper with a pinch of sea salt and black pepper to the taste and spread sesame seeds on one side.
2. Press seeds down, flip fish and spread the remaining sesame seeds on this side.
3. Heat up a pan with the oil over medium high heat, add crusted red snapper, cook for 3 minutes on each side and transfer to a plate. Serve with a side salad.

Nutrition Facts Per Serving: Calories: 120; Fat: 1; Fiber: 1; Carbs: 2; Protein: 10

Paleo Salmon And Tomato Pesto

(Prep + Cook Time: 25 minutes | Servings: 4)

Ingredients:

- 4 salmon fillets; skin on
- 1 tbsp. red bell pepper; chopped
- 1 shallot; chopped
- 2 tbsp. basil; chopped
- 1/2 cup cherry tomatoes; cut in quarters
- 2 garlic cloves; minced
- 1/2 cup sun-dried tomatoes; chopped
- 3 tbsp. olive oil
- A pinch of sea salt
- Black pepper to the taste

Instructions:

1. In your food processor, mix sun-dried tomatoes with garlic, oil, basil, shallots, a pinch of sea salt and black pepper and blend really well.
2. Rub salmon with some of this mix, place on preheated grill over medium high heat, cook for 12 minutes flipping once and divide between plates. Add the rest of the tomato pesto on top and serve with cherry tomatoes and bell pepper pieces on the side.

Nutrition Facts Per Serving: Calories: 140; Fat: 2; Fiber: 2; Carbs: 3; Protein: 9

Paleo Scallops Tartar

(Prep + Cook Time: 10 minutes | Servings: 2)

Ingredients:

- Juice of 1/2 lemon
- 1 tbsp. green onions; chopped
- 1 tbsp. olive oil
- 6 scallops; chopped
- 3 strawberries; chopped
- 1/2 tbsp. basil; chopped
- A pinch of sea salt

- Black pepper to the taste

Instructions:

1. In a bowl; mix green onions with lemon juice, olive oil, scallops, strawberries, basil, a pinch of sea salt and black pepper to the taste, stir well, divide into small bowls and serve cold.

Nutrition Facts Per Serving: Calories: 140; Fat: 2; Fiber: 2; Carbs: 3; Protein: 9

Meat Recipes

Lamb Chops With Mint Sauce

(Prep + Cook Time: 35 minutes | Servings: 4)

Ingredients:
- 2 garlic cloves; finely minced
- 8 lamb chops
- 2/3 cup extra virgin olive oil
- 1 tbsp. oregano; finely chopped
- 3 tbsp. Dijon mustard
- 1 tbsp. lemon zest
- 2 tbsp. white wine vinegar
- 1/3 cup mint; chopped
- Black pepper to the taste

Instructions:

1. In a bowl; mix olive oil with oregano, garlic and lemon zest and stir well.
2. Season lamb with black pepper to the taste and brush with the mix you've just made.
3. Heat up your grill over medium high heat, add lamb chops, cook for 5 minutes on each side and transfer to plates.

4. In a bowl; mix mustard with vinegar, pepper and mint and whisk well. Serve lamb chops with vinegar mix drizzled on top.

Nutrition Facts Per Serving: Calories: 160; Fat: 5.6; Carbs: 1; Fiber: 0.2; Protein: 23.2

Paleo Beef Kabobs

(Prep + Cook Time: 22 minutes | Servings: 4)

Ingredients:
- 2 red bell peppers; chopped
- 2 lbs. sirloin steak; cut into medium pieces
- 1 red onion; chopped
- 1 zucchini; sliced
- Juice from 1 lime
- 2 tbsp. chili powder
- 2 tbsp. hot sauce
- 1/2 tbsp. cumin powder
- 1/4 cup olive oil
- 1/4 cup Paleo Salsa
- A pinch of sea salt and black pepper to the taste

Instructions:
1. In a bowl; mix salsa with lime juice, oil, hot sauce, chili powder, cumin, salt and black pepper and whisk well.
2. Layer steaks pieces, bell peppers, zucchini and onion on skewers.
3. Brush kabobs with the salsa mix you made earlier, place them on preheated grill over medium high heat and cook them for 5 minutes on each side. Divide kabobs between plates and serve.

Nutrition Facts Per Serving: Calories: 170; Fat: 5; Fiber: 2; Carbs: 3; Protein: 8

Roasted Duck Dish

(Prep + Cook Time: 2 hours 10 minutes | Servings: 4)

Ingredients:

- 2 tsp. allspice; ground
- 4 duck legs
- 4 thyme springs
- 1 lemon; sliced
- 1 orange; sliced
- 1 cup chicken broth
- A pinch of sea salt
- Black pepper to the taste
- 1/2 cup orange juice

Instructions:

1. Heat up a pan over medium high heat, add duck legs, season with a pinch of salt and pepper to the taste and brown them for 3 minutes on each side.
2. Arrange half of lemon and orange slices on the bottom of a baking dish, place duck legs, top with the rest of the orange and lemon slices and thyme springs.
3. Add chicken stock, orange juice, sprinkle allspice, introduce in the oven at 350 °F and bake for 2 hours. Divide between plates and serve hot.

Nutrition Facts Per Serving: 255; Fat: 17; Carbs: 6; Protein: 33; Fiber: 1

Chicken Meatballs

(Prep + Cook Time: 30 minutes | Servings: 4)

Ingredients:

- 1 tsp. sweet paprika
- 1 pineapple; diced
- 1 egg

- 2 lbs. chicken meat; ground
- A pinch of sea salt
- Black pepper to the taste
- 1 tsp. garlic powder
- 1 tsp. onion powder

For the sauce:

- 1/4 cup coconut amino
- 4 tbsp. ketchup
- 1 tbsp. ginger; grated
- 1/2 cup pineapple juice
- 2 tsp. raw honey
- 1/2 tsp. red pepper flakes
- Salt and black pepper to the taste
- 1 tbsp. garlic; minced

Instructions:

1. In a pot, mix amino with ketchup, ginger, pineapple sauce, garlic, pepper flakes, honey, a pinch of sea salt and pepper to the taste, stir well, bring to a boil over medium heat, simmer for 8 minutes and take off heat.
2. In a bowl; mix chicken meat with paprika, egg, onion powder, garlic powder, salt and black pepper to the taste and stir well.
3. Shape meatballs, arrange them on a lined baking sheet, introduce them in the oven at 475 °F and bake for 15 minutes.
4. Heat up a pan over medium heat, add pineapple pieces, stir and cook for 2 minutes.
5. Add baked meatballs, pour sauce you've made at the beginnings, stir gently, cook for 5 minutes, divide between plates and serve.

Nutrition Facts Per Serving: Calories: 264; Fat: 20; Carbs: 47; Fiber: 2; Protein: 47

Paleo Beef Casserole

(Prep + Cook Time: 8 hours 10 minutes | Servings: 4)

Ingredients:

- 2 cups pearl onions
- 3½ lbs. grass fed beef meat; cubed
- 4 garlic cloves; minced
- 2 sweet potatoes; chopped
- 2 celery stalks; chopped
- A pinch of sea salt
- Black pepper to the taste
- 2 tbsp. tomato paste
- 2 bay leaves
- 2 cups carrot; chopped
- 2 cups broth
- 1 tsp. thyme; dried
- 1 tbsp. coconut oil

Instructions:

1. Heat up a pan with the oil over medium-high heat, add beef, stir and brown for 2 minutes on each side and transfer to your slow cooker.
2. Add pearl onions, potatoes, celery, garlic, carrots, tomato paste, stock, bay leaves, thyme, a pinch of salt and pepper to the taste, stir; cover and cook on Low for 8 hours. Uncover cooker, leave stew aside for 10 minutes, divide between plates and serve.

Nutrition Facts Per Serving: Calories: 210; Carbs: 14; Fat: 20; Fiber: 4; Protein: 38

Lamb Chops And Mint Sauce

(Prep + Cook Time: 30 minutes | Servings: 4)

Ingredients:

- 2 garlic cloves; minced

- 1 tbsp. lemon zest
- 1 tbsp. oregano; chopped
- 8 lamb chops
- 2/3 cup olive oil
- 1/3 cup mint; chopped
- 2 tbsp. balsamic vinegar
- A pinch of sea salt
- Black pepper to the taste
- 3 tbsp. Dijon mustard

Instructions:

1. In a bowl; mix oil with oregano, garlic and lemon zest and whisk well.
2. Brush lamb chops with this mix, season them with a pinch of salt and black pepper to the taste, place them on preheated grill over medium high heat and cook for 5 minutes on each side.
3. In a bowl; mix mustard with a pinch of salt, mint, vinegar and black pepper and whisk well. Divide lamb chops on plates, drizzle mint sauce over them and serve.

Nutrition Facts Per Serving: Calories: 17; Fat: 11; Fiber: 1; Carbs: 6; Protein: 14

Grilled Lamb Chops

(Prep + Cook Time: 20 minutes | Servings: 6)

Ingredients:

- 3 tbsp. coconut amino
- 4 tbsp. extra virgin olive oil
- 8 lamb chops
- A pinch of sea salt
- Black pepper to the taste
- 2 garlic cloves; minced
- 2 tbsp. ginger; minced

- 1 tbsp. parsley leaves; chopped

Instructions:

1. In a bowl; mix olive oil with coconut amino, garlic, ginger and parsley and stir well.
2. Season lamb chops with a pinch of sea salt and pepper to the taste, place them on preheated grill over medium-high heat and cook for 4 minutes on each side, basting all the time with the marinade you've made.
3. Divide lamb chops on plates, leave aside to cool down for 4 minutes and serve.

Nutrition Facts Per Serving: Calories: 214; Fat: 33; Carbs: 2; Protein: 28; Fiber: 0.2

Lamb Casserole

(Prep + Cook Time: 3 hours | Servings: 4)

Ingredients:

- 1 butternut squash; cubed
- 3 lbs. lamb shoulder; chopped
- 4 shallots; chopped
- 4 carrots; chopped
- 4 tomatoes; chopped
- 2 Thai chilies; chopped
- 2 tbsp. tomato paste
- 1 cinnamon stick
- 2½ cups warm beef broth
- 2-star anise
- 2 tbsp. tapioca starch
- 1 lemongrass stalk; finely chopped
- 1 tsp. Chinese five spice powder
- 1 tbsp. ginger; minced
- 2 tbsp. coconut amino
- 1½ tbsp. coconut oil
- 3 garlic cloves; chopped

- Black pepper to the taste

Instructions:

1. In a bowl; mix lamb with coconut amino, tapioca starch, ginger, lemongrass, garlic and pepper, stir well, cover and keep in the fridge for 2 hours.
2. Heat up a pot with the oil over medium-high heat, add marinated lamb, stir and brown for 3 minutes.
3. Add tomato paste and tomatoes, stir and cook for 2 more minutes.
4. Add squash, shallots, Thai chilies, carrots, cinnamon stick, star anise, beef stock and five spices, stir well, introduce in the oven at 325 °F and bake for 1 hour. Divide between plates and serve hot.

Nutrition Facts Per Serving: Calories: 456; Fat: 31; Carbs: 5; Fiber: 3; Protein: 22

Grilled Steaks

(Prep + Cook Time: 20 minutes | Servings: 4)

Ingredients:

- 1½ tbsp. coffee; ground
- 4 rib eye steaks
- 1/2 tbsp. sweet paprika
- 2 tbsp. chili powder
- 2 tsp. garlic powder
- 2 tsp. onion powder
- 1/4 tsp. ginger; ground
- 1/4 teaspoon; coriander, ground
- A pinch of cayenne pepper
- Black pepper to the taste

Instructions:

1. In a bowl; mix coffee with paprika, chili powder, garlic powder, onion powder, ginger, coriander, cayenne and black pepper and stir well.
2. Rub steaks with the coffee mix, place them on your preheated grill over medium high heat, cook them for 5 minutes on each side and divide between plates. Leave steaks to cool down for 5 minutes before serving them with a side salad!

Nutrition Facts Per Serving: Calories: 160; Fat: 10; Fiber: 1; Carbs: 4; Protein: 8

Pork Dish With Delicious Blueberry Sauce

(Prep + Cook Time: 40 minutes | Servings: 4)

Ingredients:
- 1 cup blueberries
- 1/2 tsp. thyme; dried
- 2 lbs. pork loin
- 1 tbsp. balsamic vinegar
- 1/2 tsp. red chili flakes
- 1 tsp. ginger powder
- A pinch of sea salt
- Black pepper to the taste
- **2 tbsp. water**

Instructions:
1. Put pork loin in a baking dish and season with a pinch of sea salt and pepper to the taste.
2. Heat up a pan over medium heat, add blueberries and mix with vinegar, water, thyme, chili flakes and ginger.
3. Stir well, cook for 5 minutes and pour over pork loin. Introduce in the oven at 375 °F and bake for 25 minutes.
4. Take pork out of the oven, leave aside for 5 minutes, slice, divide between plates and serve with blueberries sauce.

Nutrition Facts Per Serving: Calories: 325; Fat: 23; Carbs: 6; Fiber: 1; Protein: 64

Paleo Pulled Pork

(Prep + Cook Time: 20 hours 30 minutes | Servings: 4)

Ingredients:

- 1/2 cup salsa
- 1/2 cup beef stock
- 1/2 cup enchilada sauce
- 3 lbs. organic pork shoulder
- 2 green chilies; chopped
- 1 tbsp. garlic powder
- 1 tbsp. chili powder
- 1 tsp. onion powder
- 1 tsp. cumin
- 1 tsp. paprika
- Black pepper to the taste

Instructions:

1. In a bowl; mix chili powder with onion and garlic one.
2. Add cumin, paprika and pepper to the taste and stir everything.
3. Add pork, rub well and keep in the fridge for 12 hours.
4. Transfer pork to your slow cooker, add enchilada sauce, stock, salsa and green chilies, stir; cover and cook on Low for 8 hours.
5. Transfer pork to a plate, leave aside to cool down and shred.
6. Strain sauce from slow cooker into a pan, bring to a boil over medium heat and simmer for 8 minutes stirring all the time.
7. Add shredded pork to the sauce, stir; reduce heat to medium and cook for 20 more minutes. Divide between plates and serve hot.

Nutrition Facts Per Serving: Calories: 250; Fat: 35; Carbs: 5; Fiber: 2; Protein: 50

Beef Lasagna

(Prep + Cook Time: 6 hours 10 minutes | Servings: 6)

Ingredients:

- 1 red bell pepper; chopped
- 1 eggplant; sliced lengthwise
- 2 zucchinis; sliced lengthwise
- 1 lb. beef; ground
- 2 cups tomatoes; chopped
- 2 tsp. oregano; dried
- 4 cups tomato sauce
- 1/4 cup basil; chopped
- 2 garlic cloves; minced
- 1 yellow onion; chopped
- 2 tbsp. tomato paste
- 1 tbsp. parsley; chopped
- 2 tbsp. olive oil
- A pinch of sea salt
- Black pepper to the taste

Instructions:

1. Heat up a pan with the oil over medium high heat, add onion and garlic, stir and cook for 2 minutes.
2. Add beef, stir and brown for 5 minutes more.
3. Add bell pepper, tomatoes, oregano, basil, tomato paste and parsley, stir and cook for 4 minutes more.
4. Add tomato sauce, black pepper to the taste and a pinch of salt and stir well again.
5. Arrange layers of eggplant and zucchini slices with the sauce you've made in your slow cooker.
6. Cover and cook on Low for 4 hours and 45 minutes. Divide your lasagna between plates and serve.

Nutrition Facts Per Serving: Calories: 240; Fat: 10; Fiber: 5; Carbs: 7; Protein: 12

Pork With Pear Salsa

(Prep + Cook Time: 55 minutes | Servings: 4)

Ingredients:

- 1 yellow onion; chopped
- 1 organic pork tenderloin
- 2 pears; chopped
- 2 garlic cloves; minced
- 1 tbsp. chives; chopped
- 1/4 cup walnuts; chopped
- 3 tbsp. balsamic vinegar
- Black pepper to the taste
- 1/2 cup chicken stock
- 1 tbsp. coconut oil
- 1 tbsp. lemon juice

Instructions:

1. In a bowl; mix walnuts with pear, chives, pepper and lemon juice and stir well.
2. Heat up a pan with the oil over medium high heat, add tenderloin and brown for 3 minutes on each side.
3. Reduce heat, add onion and garlic, stir and cook for 2 minutes. Add balsamic vinegar, stock, pear mix, stir; introduce in the oven at 400 °F and bake for 20 minutes.
4. Take pork out of the oven, leave aside for 4 minutes, slice, divide between plates and serve with pear salsa on top.

Nutrition Facts Per Serving: Calories: 170; Fat: 3; Carbs: 19; Fiber: 4.4; Sugar: 10; Protein: 12

Turkey Casserole

(Prep + Cook Time: 1 hour 10 minutes | Servings: 6)

Ingredients:

- 1 sweet potato; chopped
- 1 lb. turkey meat; ground
- 1 eggplant; thinly sliced
- 1 yellow onion; finely chopped
- 1 tbsp. garlic; finely minced
- A pinch of sea salt
- Black pepper to the taste
- 1/4 tsp. chili powder
- 1/4 tsp. cumin
- 15 oz. canned tomatoes; chopped and drained
- 8 oz. tomato paste
- A drizzle of olive oil
- 1/2 tsp. tarragon flakes
- 1/8 tsp. cardamom; ground
- 1/8 tsp. oregano

For the sauce:

- 1 tbsp. almond flour
- 1 cup almond milk
- 1½ tbsp. extra virgin olive oil
- 1 tbsp. coconut flour

Instructions:

1. Heat up a pan over medium-high heat, add turkey meat, onion and garlic, stir and cook until the meat turns brown.
2. Add tomatoes, tomato paste and sweet potatoes, stir and cook for 5 minutes.
3. Add a pinch of sea salt, pepper to the taste, chili powder, cumin, oregano, tarragon flakes and cardamom, stir well and cook for 2 minutes.
4. Grease a baking dish with a drizzle of olive oil, arrange eggplant slices on the bottom and add turkey mix on top.

94

5. Spread turkey mix evenly, introduce dish in the oven at 350 °F and bake for 15 minutes.
6. Meanwhile; heat up a pot over medium-high heat, add the rest of the olive oil, almond flour and coconut one, stir well 1 minute, reduce heat, add almond milk and stir well.
7. Cook this for 10 minutes.
8. Take the baking dish out of the oven and pour this almond milk mix over it.
9. Introduce in the oven again and bake for 45 minutes. Take casserole out of the oven, leave aside a few minutes to cool down, slice and divide between plates and serve.

Nutrition Facts Per Serving: Calories: 278; Fat: 2.6; Carbs: 29; Fiber: 6.7; Sugar: 13; Protein: 28.5

Chicken Thighs With Tasty Squash

(Prep + Cook Time: 40 minutes | Servings: 6)

Ingredients:

- 6 chicken thighs; boneless and skinless
- 1/2 lb. bacon; chopped
- 2 tbsp. coconut oil
- A pinch of sea salt
- A handful sage; chopped
- Black pepper to the taste
- 3 cups butternut squash; cubed

Instructions:

1. Heat up a pan over medium heat, add bacon, cook until it's crispy, drain on paper towels, transfer to a plate, crumble and leave aside for now.
2. Heat up the same pan over medium heat, add butternut squash, a pinch of salt and black pepper to the taste, stir; cook until it's soft, transfer to a plate and also leave aside.

3. Heat up the pan again with the coconut oil over medium-high heat, add chicken, salt and pepper and cook for 10 minutes, turning often.
4. Take the pan off the heat, add squash, introduce in the oven at 425 °F and bake for 15 minutes. Divide chicken and butternut on plates, top with sage and bacon and serve.

Nutrition Facts Per Serving: Calories: 241; Fat: 11; Carbs: 17; Fiber: 2.5; Sugar: 3; Protein: 16

Stuffed Quail

(Prep + Cook Time: 1 hour 15 minutes | Servings: 4)

Ingredients:
- 8 bacon slices
- 4 quails
- 1 apple; chopped
- 1 lb. grapes
- 1 tbsp. rosemary; chopped
- 1/2 cup cranberries; chopped
- 2 tbsp. extra virgin olive oil
- 2 garlic cloves; chopped
- 4 rosemary springs
- 1/2 cup chicken stock
- A pinch of sea salt
- Black pepper to the taste

Instructions:
1. Pat dry quail, season with a pinch of sea salt and pepper and leave aside for now.
2. In a bowl; mix cranberries with chopped rosemary, apple, olive oil, garlic, salt and pepper to the taste and stir well.
3. Fill quail with this mix, wrap each with 2 bacon slices and tie with cooking twine.

4. Spread half of the grapes in a baking dish, mash gently with a fork, arrange quail on top, spread the rest of the grapes and pour chicken stock at the end.
5. Introduce everything in the oven at 425 °F and bake for 1 hour. Divide between plates and serve with baked grapes on the side.

Nutrition Facts Per Serving: Calories: 260; Fat: 18; Carbs: 22; Fiber: 3; Protein: 29

Delicious Paleo Steak

(Prep + Cook Time: 40 minutes | Servings: 4)

Ingredients:
- 2 sweet potatoes; chopped
- 4 sirloin steaks
- 1 red onion; chopped
- 1 broccoli head; florets separated
- 8 cherry tomatoes; halved
- 4 thyme springs
- 4 garlic cloves; minced
- A pinch of sea salt
- Black pepper to the taste
- 4 tbsp. olive oil
- 1/2 tbsp. sweet paprika

Instructions:
1. In a bowl; mix oil with a pinch of salt, black pepper, garlic and paprika and stir well.
2. Spread broccoli and sweet potatoes on a lined baking sheet, place in the oven at 425 degrees f and bake for 10 minutes.
3. Heat up a pan over medium high heat, add steaks, season them with a pinch of sea salt and black pepper, cook for 2 minutes on each side and add to the baking sheet.

4. Also add onions and tomatoes, drizzle the oil and garlic mix, toss to coat, top with thyme and bake in the oven for 15 minutes more. Divide everything between plates and serve.

Nutrition Facts Per Serving: Calories: 170; Fat: 2; Fiber: 2; Carbs: 4; Protein: 10

Paleo Beef And Bok Choy

(Prep + Cook Time: 30 minutes | Servings: 4)

Ingredients:

- 1 onion; sliced
- 12 baby bok choy heads; halved
- 2 lb. beef sirloin; cut into strips
- 2 garlic cloves; minced
- 3 tbsp. coconut oil
- 5 red chilies; dried and chopped
- A pinch of sea salt
- Black pepper to the taste
- 1 ginger piece; grated

Instructions:

1. Heat up a pan with the oil over high heat, add chilies, garlic and ginger, stir and cook for 1 minute.
2. Add beef, stir; cook for 3 minutes and transfer to a bowl.
3. Heat up the pan again over medium high heat, add onion, stir and cook for 2 minutes.
4. Add bok choy, stir and cook for 4 minutes more. Return beef mix to the pan, stir; cook for 1 minute more, divide between plates and serve hot.

Nutrition Facts Per Serving: Calories: 140; Fat: 3; Fiber: 5; Carbs: 9; Protein: 20

Paleo Chicken And Veggies Stir Fry

(Prep + Cook Time: 35 minutes | Servings: 4)

Ingredients:

- 1 red bell pepper; chopped
- 1 zucchini; chopped
- 1 yellow onion; finely chopped
- 1 broccoli head; florets separated
- 4 chicken breasts; skinless, boneless and chopped
- A pinch of sea salt
- Black pepper to the taste
- 1 tbsp. coconut oil

For the sauce:

- 1/4 cup chicken broth
- 2 garlic cloves; finely chopped
- 3 tbsp. coconut amino
- 1/2 cup orange juice
- 1 tbsp. orange zest
- 1 tsp. Sriracha sauce
- 1/4 tsp. ginger; grated
- A pinch of red pepper flakes

Instructions:

1. In a bowl; mix broth with orange juice, zest, amino, ginger, garlic, pepper flakes and Sriracha sauce and stir well.
2. Heat up a pan with the oil over medium heat, add chicken, cook for 8 minutes and transfer to a plate.
3. Heat up the same pan over medium heat, add bell pepper, broccoli florets, onion and zucchini, stir and cook for 4-5 minutes.
4. Add a pinch of sea salt, pepper, orange sauce you've made, stir; bring to a boil, add chicken, reduce heat and simmer for 8 minutes. Divide between plates and serve hot.

Nutrition Facts Per Serving: Calories: 320; Fat: 13; Carbs: 17; Protein: 45; Fiber: 3.7; Sugar: 4

Sausage Casserole

(Prep + Cook Time: 60 minutes | Servings: 6)

Ingredients:

- 6 sausage
- 2 green bell peppers; chopped
- 3 sweet potatoes; chopped
- 1-pint grape tomatoes; chopped
- A pinch of sea salt
- Black pepper to the taste
- 2 garlic cloves; minced
- 1 red onion; chopped
- A few thyme springs

Instructions:

1. In a baking dish, mix potatoes with tomatoes, onion, bell pepper, garlic, a pinch of sea salt and pepper and stir gently.
2. Heat up a pan over high heat, add sausages, brown them for 2 minutes on each side and transfer on top of veggies in the baking dish.
3. Add thyme, introduce in the oven at 400 °F and bake for 45 minutes. Divide between plates and serve hot.

Nutrition Facts Per Serving: Calories: 355; Fat: 10; Carbs: 25; Fiber: 2; Protein: 16

Paleo Steaks And Apricots

(Prep + Cook Time: 35 minutes | Servings: 2)

Ingredients:

- 2 tbsp. Cajun spice
- 1/4 cup coconut oil
- 2 medium skirt steaks
- 1/3 cup lemon juice
- 1/4 cup apricot preserves

- 1/4 cup coconut aminos

Instructions:

1. In a bowl; mix half of the Cajun spice with lemon juice, aminos, oil and apricot preserves and stir well.
2. Pour this into a pan, bring to a boil over medium high heat and simmer for 8 minutes.
3. Blend this using an immersion blender and leave aside for now.
4. Season steaks with the rest of the Cajun spice, brush them with half of the apricots mix, place them on preheated grill over medium high heat and cook them for 6-minute son each side. Divide steaks on plates and top with the rest of the apricots mix.

Nutrition Facts Per Serving: Calories: 160; Fat: 6; Fiber: 0.1; Carbs: 1; Protein: 22

Beef Tenderloin With Special Sauce

(Prep + Cook Time: 50 minutes | Servings: 4) Ingredients:

- 3 tbsp. Dijon mustard
- 3 lbs. beef tenderloin
- A pinch of sea salt
- Black pepper to the taste
- 1 tbsp. coconut oil
- 3 tbsp. balsamic vinegar

For the sauce:
- 3 tbsp. basil leaves; chopped
- 1/2 cup parsley leaves; chopped
- Zest from 1 lemon
- 2 garlic cloves; finely chopped
- A pinch of sea salt

- Black pepper to the taste
- 1/4 cup extra virgin olive oil

Instructions:

1. In a bowl; mix mustard with vinegar, stir very well and leave aside.
2. Season beef with a pinch of sea salt and pepper to the taste put in a pan heated with the coconut oil over medium-high heat and cook for 2 minutes on each side.
3. Transfer beef to a baking pan, cover with the mustard mix, introduce in the oven at 475 °F and bake for 25 minutes.
4. Meanwhile; in a bowl, mix parsley with basil, lemon zest, garlic, olive oil, a pinch of sea salt and pepper to the taste and whisk very well.
5. Take beef tenderloin out if the oven, leave aside for a few minutes to cool down, slice and divide between plates. Serve with herbs sauce on the side.

Nutrition Facts Per Serving: Calories: 180; Fat: 13; Carbs: 2; Fiber: 2; Protein: 7

Paleo Steaks And Scallops

(Prep + Cook Time: 30 minutes | Servings: 2)

Ingredients:
- 10 sea scallops
- 4 garlic cloves; minced
- 2 beef steaks
- 1 shallot; chopped
- 2 tbsp. lemon juice
- 2 tbsp. parsley; chopped
- 2 tbsp. basil; chopped
- 1 tsp. lemon zest
- 1/4 cup ghee
- 1/4 cup veggie stock

- Some bacon fat
- A pinch of sea salt
- Black pepper to the taste

Instructions:

1. Heat up a pan with some bacon fat over medium high heat, add steaks, season them with a pinch of salt and black pepper to the taste and cook for 4 minutes on each side.
2. Add shallot and garlic, stir and cook for 2 minutes more.
3. Add ghee and stir everything.
4. Add stock, basil, lemon juice, parsley and lemon zest and stir.
5. Add scallops, season them with some black pepper as well and cook for a couple more minutes. Divide steaks and scallops between plates and serve with pan juices.

Nutrition Facts Per Serving: Calories: 150; Fat: 2; Fiber: 2; Carbs: 4; Protein: 14

Beef Stir Fry

(Prep + Cook Time: 30 minutes | Servings: 4)

Ingredients:

- 10 oz. mushrooms; sliced
- 10 oz. asparagus; sliced
- 1½ lbs. beef steak; thinly sliced
- 2 tbsp. honey
- 1/3 cup coconut amino
- 2 tsp. apple cider vinegar
- 1/2 tsp. ginger; minced
- 6 garlic cloves; minced
- 1 chili; sliced
- 1 tbsp. coconut oil
- Black pepper to the taste

Instructions:

1. In a bowl; mix garlic with coconut amino, honey, ginger and vinegar and whisk well.
2. Put some water in a pan, heat up over medium high heat, add asparagus and black pepper, cook for 3 minutes, transfer to a bowl filled with ice water, drain and leave aside.
3. Heat up a pan with the oil over medium-high heat, add mushrooms, cook for 2 minutes on each side, transfer to a bowl and also leave aside.
4. Heat up the same pan over high heat, add meat, brown for a few minutes and mix with chili pepper.
5. Cook for 2 more minutes and mix with asparagus, mushrooms and vinegar sauce you've made at the beginning. Stir well, cook for 3 minutes, take off heat, divide between plates and serve.

Nutrition Facts Per Serving: Calories: 165; Fat: 7.2; Carbs: 6.33; Fiber: 1.3; Sugar: 3; Protein: 18.4

Barbeque Ribs

(Prep + Cook Time: 3 hour 2 minutes | Servings: 4)

Ingredients:
- 1 tbsp. smoked paprika
- 1/2 tbsp. onion powder
- 1/2 tbsp. garlic powder
- 1/2 tsp. cayenne pepper
- 4 lbs. baby ribs
- 1 cup paleo BBQ sauce
- 2 tbsp. raw honey
- 4 tsp. Sriracha
- 1/4 cup cilantro; chopped
- 1/4 cup chives; chopped
- 1/4 cup parsley; chopped
- Black pepper to the taste

Instructions:

1. In a bowl; mix paprika with onion powder, garlic powder, pepper and cayenne and stir well.
2. Add ribs, toss to coat and arrange them on a lined baking sheet.
3. Introduce in the oven at 325 °F and bake them for 2 hours and 30 minutes.
4. In a bowl; mix BBQ sauce with honey and Sriracha and stir well.
5. Take ribs out of the oven, mix them with BBQ sauce, place them on preheated grill over medium-high heat and cook for 7 minutes on each side. Divide ribs on plates, sprinkle chives, cilantro and parsley on top and serve.

Nutrition Facts Per Serving: Calories: 120; Fat: 6.4; Carbs: 2; Fiber: 03; Sugar: 0.3; Protein: 6.2

Paleo Pork Chops

(Prep + Cook Time: 40 minutes | Servings: 4)

Ingredients:
- 8 sage springs
- 4 pork chops; bone-in
- 4 tbsp. ghee
- 4 garlic cloves; crushed
- 1 tbsp. coconut oil
- A pinch of sea salt
- Black pepper to the taste

Instructions:

1. Season pork chops with a pinch of sea salt and pepper to the taste.
2. Heat up a pan with the oil over medium high heat, add pork chops and cook for 10 minutes turning them often.

3. Take pork chops off heat, add ghee, sage and garlic and toss to coat. Return to heat, cook for 4 minutes often stirring, divide between plates and serve.

Nutrition Facts Per Serving: Calories: 250; Fat: 41; Carbs: 1; Fiber: 1; Sugar: 0.1; Protein: 18.3

Pork Tenderloin With Carrot Puree

(Prep + Cook Time: 55 minutes | Servings: 4)

Ingredients:

- 2 sausages; casings removed
- A handful arugula
- Black pepper to the taste
- 1 grass fed pork tenderloin
- 1 tbsp. coconut oil

For the puree:

- 1 sweet potato; chopped
- 3 carrots; chopped
- A pinch of sea salt
- Black pepper to the taste
- 1 tbsp. curry paste

For the sauce:

- 2 tbsp. balsamic vinegar
- 1 tsp. mustard
- 2 shallots; finely chopped
- Black pepper to the taste
- 4 tbsp. extra virgin olive oil

Instructions:

1. Slice pork tenderloin in half horizontally but not all the way and open it up.
2. Use a meat tenderizer to even it up.
3. Place sausage in the middle, roll pork around it, tie with twine, season pepper to the taste and leave aside.

4. Heat up an oven proof pan with the coconut oil over medium high heat, add pork roll, cook for 3 minutes on each side, introduce in the oven at 350 °F and bake for 25 minutes.
5. Meanwhile; put potatoes and carrots in a pot, add water to cover, bring to a boil over medium high heat, cook for 20 minutes, drain and transfer to your food processor.
6. Pulse a few times until you obtain a puree, add a pinch of sea salt and pepper to the taste, blend again, transfer to a bowl and leave aside.
7. Take pork roll out of the oven, slice and divide between plates.
8. Heat up a pan with the olive oil over medium high heat, add shallots, stir and cook for 10 minutes.
9. Add balsamic vinegar, mustard, pepper, stir well and take off heat. Divide carrots puree next to pork slices, drizzle vinegar sauce on to and serve with arugula on the side.

Nutrition Facts Per Serving: Calories: 250; Fat: 34; Carbs: 19; Fiber: 2; Protein: 53

Pork With Strawberry Sauce

(Prep + Cook Time: 45 minutes | Servings: 4)

Ingredients:
- 4 lbs. pork tenderloin
- 1 cup strawberries; sliced
- 10 bacon slices
- A pinch of sea salt
- Black pepper to the taste
- 4 garlic cloves; minced
- 1/2 cup balsamic vinegar
- 2 tbsp. extra virgin olive oil

Instructions:

1. Wrap bacon slices around tenderloin, secure with toothpicks and season with salt and pepper.
2. Heat up your grill over indirect medium high heat, put tenderloin on it and cook for 30 minutes.
3. Heat up a pan with the oil over medium high heat, add garlic, stir and cook for 2 minutes.
4. Add vinegar and half of the strawberries, stir and bring to a boil.
5. Reduce heat to medium and simmer for 10 minutes.
6. Add black pepper to the taste and the rest of the strawberries and stir.
7. Baste pork with some of the sauce and continue cooking over indirect heat until bacon is crispy enough.
8. Transfer pork to a cutting board, leave aside for a few minutes to cool down, slice and divide between plates. Serve with the strawberry sauce right away.

Nutrition Facts Per Serving: Calories: 279; Fat: 30; Carbs: 8; Fiber: 22; Protein: 125

Paleo Souvlaki

(Prep + Cook Time: 30 minutes | Servings: 4)
Ingredients:
- 3 sweet potatoes; cubed
- 1 yellow onion; chopped
- 12 mini bell peppers; chopped
- 4 medium round steaks
- 1/2 cup sun dried tomatoes; chopped
- 1 tbsp. sweet paprika
- 2 tbsp. balsamic vinegar
- Juice of 1 lemon
- 1 tbsp. oregano; dried
- 1/4 cup olive oil
- 1 lemon; sliced
- 1/4 cup kalamata olives; pitted and chopped

- 4 dill springs
- 2 garlic cloves; minced
- Some bacon fat
- A pinch of sea salt and black pepper

Instructions:

1. Heat up a pan with some bacon fat over medium high heat, add steaks, season them with a pinch of sea salt and some black pepper, brown them for 2 minutes on each side and transfer to a baking dish.
2. Heat up the pan again over medium high heat, add sweet potatoes, cook them for 4 minutes and add them to the baking dish.
3. Also add bell peppers, tomatoes, onion, olives and lemon slices.
4. Meanwhile; in a bowl, mix lemon juice with olive oil, vinegar, garlic, paprika and oregano and whisk well.
5. Pour this over steak and veggies, add dill springs on top, toss to coat, place in the oven at 425 °F and bake for 12 minutes. Divide steak and veggies between plates and serve.

Nutrition Facts Per Serving: Calories: 180; Fat: 11; Fiber: 0; Carbs: 0; Protein: 21

Mexican Steaks

(Prep + Cook Time: 25 minutes | Servings: 4)

Ingredients:

- 2 tbsp. chili powder
- 4 medium sirloin steaks
- 1 tsp. cumin; ground
- 1/2 tbsp. sweet paprika
- 1 tsp. onion powder
- 1 tsp. garlic powder
- A pinch of sea salt and black pepper to the taste

For the Pico de gallo:
- 1 small red onion; chopped
- 2 tomatoes; chopped
- 2 garlic cloves; minced
- 2 tbsp. lime juice
- 1 small green bell pepper; chopped
- 1 jalapeno; chopped
- 1/4 cup cilantro; chopped
- 1/4 tsp. cumin; ground
- Black pepper to the taste

Instructions:

1. In a bowl; mix chili powder with a pinch of salt, black pepper, onion powder, garlic powder, paprika and 1 tsp. cumin and stir well.
2. Season steaks with this mix, rub well and place them on preheated grill over medium high heat.
3. Cook steaks for 5 minutes on each side and divide them between plates.
4. In a bowl; mix red onion with tomatoes, garlic, lime juice, bell pepper, jalapeno, cilantro, black pepper to the taste and 1/4 tsp. cumin and stir well. Top steaks with this mix and serve.

Nutrition Facts Per Serving: Calories: 200; Fat: 12; Fiber: 4; Carbs: 5; Protein: 12

Paleo Moroccan Lamb

(Prep + Cook Time: 17 minutes | Servings: 4)

Ingredients:
- 8 lamb chops
- 2 tbsp. ras el hanout
- 1 tsp. olive oil

For the sauce:

- 1/4 cup parsley; chopped
- 2 tbsp. mint; chopped
- 3 garlic cloves; minced
- 2 tbsp. lemon zest
- 1/4 cup olive oil
- 1/2 tsp. smoked paprika
- 1 tsp. red pepper flakes
- 2 tbsp. lemon juice
- A pinch of sea salt
- Black pepper to the taste

Instructions:

1. Rub lamb chops with ras el hanout and 1 tsp. oil, place them on preheated grill over medium high heat, cook them for 2 minutes on each side and divide them between plates.
2. In your food processor, mix parsley with mint, garlic, lemon zest, 1/4 cup oil, paprika, pepper flakes, lemon juice, a pinch of salt and black pepper and pulse really well. Drizzle this over lamb chops and serve.

Nutrition Facts Per Serving: Calories: 400; Fat: 23; Fiber: 1; Carbs: 3; Protein: 32

Paleo Sheppard's Pie

(Prep + Cook Time: 60 minutes | Servings: 6)

Ingredients:

- 2 lbs. sweet potatoes; chopped
- 1½ lbs. beef; ground
- 2 cups beef stock
- 1 onion; chopped
- 2 carrots; chopped
- 2 thyme springs
- 2 bay leaves
- 2 garlic cloves; minced

- 2 celery stalks; chopped
- 1/4 cup ghee
- Bacon fat
- A handful parsley; chopped
- 2 tbsp. tomato paste
- A pinch of sea salt
- Black pepper to the taste

Instructions:

1. Put sweet potatoes in a pot, add water to cover, bring to a boil over medium high heat, cook for 20 minutes, drain, leave them to cool down and transfer to a bowl.
2. Add ghee, a pinch of salt and pepper and mash potatoes well.
3. Heat up a pan with the bacon fat over medium high heat, add beef, stir and cook for a couple of minutes.
4. Add carrots, garlic, onions, celery, stock, tomato paste, bay leaves, thyme springs, some black pepper and another pinch of salt, stir and cook for 10 minutes.
5. Discard bay leaves and thyme and spread beef mix on the bottom of a baking dish.
6. Top with mashed potatoes, spread well, place in the oven at 375 °F and bake for 25 minutes. Leave pie to cool down a bit before slicing and serving it.

Nutrition Facts Per Serving: Calories: 254; Fat: 7; Fiber: 4; Carbs: 7; Protein: 14

Filet Mignon And Special Sauce

(Prep + Cook Time: 35 minutes | Servings: 4)

Ingredients:

- 12 mushrooms; sliced
- 1 shallot; chopped
- 4 fillet mignons
- 2 garlic cloves; minced

- 2 tbsp. olive oil
- 1/4 cup Dijon mustard
- 1/4 cup wine
- 1¼ cup coconut cream
- 2 tbsp. parsley; chopped
- Black pepper to the taste
- A pinch of sea salt

Instructions:

1. Heat up a pan with the oil over medium high heat, add garlic and shallots, stir and cook for 3 minutes.
2. Add mushrooms, stir and cook for 4 minutes more.
3. Add wine, stir and cook until it evaporates.
4. Add coconut cream, mustard, parsley, a pinch of salt and black pepper to the taste, stir and cook for 6 minutes more.
5. Heat up another pan over high heat, add fillets, season them with a pinch of salt and some black pepper and cook them for 4 minutes on each side. Divide fillets between plates and serve with the mushroom sauce on top.

Nutrition Facts Per Serving: Calories: 300; Fat: 12; Fiber: 1; Carbs: 4; Protein: 23

Paleo Veal Rolls

(Prep + Cook Time: 30 minutes | Servings: 4)
Ingredients:
- 2 zucchinis; cut in quarters
- 8 veal scallops
- 2 tbsp. olive oil
- 2 tsp. garlic powder
- 1/4 cup balsamic vinegar
- A pinch of sea salt
- Black pepper to the taste

Instructions:

1. Flatten veal scallops with a meat tenderizer, season them with a pinch of sea salt and black pepper to the taste and leave aside.
2. Season zucchini with a pinch of sea salt, black pepper and garlic powder, place on preheated grill over medium high heat, cook for 2 minutes on each side and transfer to a working surface.
3. Roll veal around each zucchini piece.
4. In a bowl; mix oil with balsamic vinegar and whisk well.
5. Brush veal rolls with this mix, place them on your grill and cook for 3 minutes on each side. Serve right away.

Nutrition Facts Per Serving: Calories: 160; Fat: 3; Fiber: 2; Carbs: 5; Protein: 14

Paleo Beef Teriyaki

(Prep + Cook Time: 30 minutes | Servings: 4)

Ingredients:

- 2 green onions; chopped
- 1½ lbs. steaks; sliced
- 1/4 cup honey
- 1/2 cup coconut aminos
- 1 tbsp. ginger; minced
- 1 tbsp. tapioca flour
- 1 tbsp. water
- 2 garlic cloves; minced
- 1/4 cup pear juice
- Some bacon fat
- 4 tbsp. white wine

Instructions:

1. Heat up a pan with the bacon fat over medium heat, add ginger and garlic, stir and cook for 2 minutes.
2. Add wine, stir and cook until it evaporates.

3. Add honey, aminos, pear juice, stir; bring to a simmer and cook for 12 minutes.
4. Add tapioca mixed with the water, stir and cook until it thickens.
5. Heat up a pan with some bacon fat over medium high heat, add steak slices and brown them for 2 minutes on each side.
6. Add green onions and half of the sauce you've just made, stir gently and cook for 3 minutes more. Divide steaks between plates and serve with the rest of the sauce on top.

Nutrition Facts Per Serving: Calories: 170; Fat: 3; Fiber: 2; Carbs: 2; Protein: 8

Beef And Wonderful Gravy

(Prep + Cook Time: 30 minutes | Servings: 4)

Ingredients:
- 1 egg; whisked
- 1 tbsp. mustard
- 1 tbsp. tomato paste
- 1 tsp. garlic powder
- 1 tsp. onion powder
- Some coconut oil for cooking
- A pinch of sea salt and black pepper to the taste
- 1½ lb. beef; ground

For the gravy:
- 2 tsp. parsley; chopped
- 2 tbsp. ghee
- 1 tsp. tapioca
- 1 small yellow onion; chopped
- 1¼ cups beef stock
- Black pepper to the taste

Instructions:

1. In a bowl; mix beef with tomato paste, egg, mustard, onion powder, garlic powder, a pinch of salt and black pepper to the taste and stir well.
2. Heat up a pan with the ghee over medium heat, add onion, stir and cook for 2 minutes.
3. Add stock, some black pepper, tapioca mixed with water, stir; cook until it thickens and take off heat.
4. Shape 4 patties from the beef mix. Heat up a pan with the coconut oil over medium high heat, add beef patties and cook for 5 minutes on each side.
5. Pour the gravy over beef patties, sprinkle parsley on top, cook for a couple more minutes, divide between plates and serve.

Nutrition Facts Per Serving: Calories: 200; Fat: 4; Fiber: 2; Carbs: 4; Protein: 20

Paleo Turkey Casserole

(Prep + Cook Time: 1 hour 10 minutes | Servings: 6)

Ingredients:

- 1/4 cup onion; chopped
- 1 lb. turkey meat; ground
- 1 sweet potato; cut with a spiralizer
- 1 eggplant; chopped
- 1 tbsp. garlic; minced
- 8 oz. tomato paste
- 15 oz. canned tomatoes; chopped
- A pinch of sea salt
- Black pepper to the taste
- A pinch of oregano; dried
- 1/4 tsp. chili powder
- 1/4 tsp. cumin; ground
- Cooking spray
- A pinch of cardamom; ground
- 1/2 tsp. tarragon flakes

For the sauce:

- 1 tbsp. coconut flour
- 1 tbsp. almond flour
- 1 cup almond milk
- 1½ tbsp. olive oil

Instructions:

1. Heat up a pan over medium heat, add onion, turkey and garlic, stir and brown for a few minutes.
2. Add tomatoes, tomato paste and sweet potatoes, stir and cook for a few minutes more.
3. In a bowl; mix eggplant pieces with a pinch of sea salt, black pepper, chili powder, cumin, oregano, cardamom and tarragon flakes and stir well.
4. Spread eggplant into a baking dish after you sprayed it with some cooking spray and top with the turkey mix.

5. Place in the oven at 350 °F and bake for 15 minutes.
6. Meanwhile; heat up a pan with the oil over medium heat, add coconut and almond flour and stir for 1 minute.
7. Add almond milk and cook for 10 minutes stirring often.
8. Top turkey casserole with this sauce, place in the oven again and bake for 40 minutes more. Slice and serve hot.

Nutrition Facts Per Serving: Calories: 278; Fat: 3; Fiber: 7; Carbs: 9; Protein: 18

Paleo Lamb Chops

(Prep + Cook Time: 20 minutes | Servings: 6)

Ingredients:
- 3 tbsp. coconut aminos
- 4 tbsp. olive oil
- 2 tbsp. ginger; grated
- 8 lamb chops
- 1 tbsp. parsley; chopped
- 2 garlic cloves; minced
- A pinch of sea salt
- Black pepper to the taste

Instructions:
1. In a bowl; mix oil with aminos, parsley, ginger and garlic and stir well.
2. Place lamb chops on a preheated grill over medium high heat, season them with a pinch of salt and black pepper to the taste and grill them for 4 minutes on each side basting them with the oil and ginger mix you've made. Leave lamb chops to cool down for a couple of minutes and then serve.

Nutrition Facts Per Serving: Calories: 160; Fat: 5; Fiber: 0; Carbs: 1; Protein: 20

Paleo Carne Asada

(Prep + Cook Time: 55 minutes | Servings: 2)

Ingredients:

- 1/4 cup olive oil
- 1/2 tsp. oregano; dried
- 2 garlic cloves; minced
- Juice from 1 lime
- 2 skirt steaks
- 1/4 tsp. cumin; ground
- 1 Serrano chili pepper; minced
- 1/4 cup cilantro; chopped
- A pinch of sea salt
- Black pepper to the taste

For the veggie mix:

- 2 red bell peppers; chopped
- 3 Portobello mushrooms; sliced
- 1 yellow onion; chopped
- 1 tbsp. olive oil
- 1 tbsp. lime juice
- 1 tbsp. taco seasoning

Instructions:

1. In a bowl; mix 1/4 cup oil with oregano, garlic, lime juice, cumin, cilantro, chili pepper, a pinch of salt and black pepper and whisk very well.
2. Add steaks, toss to coat and keep in the fridge for 30 minutes.
3. Place steaks on preheated grill over medium high heat, cook them for 4 minutes on each side and transfer to a plate.
4. Heat up a pan with 1 tbsp. oil over medium high heat, add bell pepper and onion, stir and cook for 3 minutes,
5. Add mushrooms, taco seasoning and lime juice, stir and cook for 6 minutes more. Divide steaks between plates and serve with mixed veggies on the side.

Nutrition Facts Per Serving: Calories: 190; Fat: 2; Fiber: 1; Carbs: 4; Protein: 20

Paleo Slow-Cooked Beef

(Prep + Cook Time: 8 hours 50 minutes | Servings: 4)

Ingredients:

- 2 cups beef stock
- 1/4 cup honey
- 1 cup tomato paste
- 1 cup balsamic vinegar
- 4 lbs. beef chuck
- 1 tbsp. mustard
- 1 tbsp. sweet paprika
- 1 tsp. onion powder
- 2 tbsp. chili powder
- 2 garlic cloves; minced
- Black pepper to the taste

Instructions:

1. In a bowl; mix beef chuck with chili powder, paprika, onion powder, garlic and black pepper and rub well.
2. Transfer beef roast to your slow cooker, add stock over it, cover and cook on Low for 8 hours.
3. Meanwhile; heat up a pan over medium heat, add tomato paste, vinegar, mustard, honey and black pepper, stir; bring to a boil and cook for 12 minutes.
4. Transfer beef roast to a cutting board, leave it to cool down a bit, shred with a fork and return to your crock pot.
5. Add the sauce you've made in the pan, cover and cook everything on High for 30 minutes more. Divide this whole mix between plates and serve.

Nutrition Facts Per Serving: Calories: 340; Fat: 5; Fiber: 2; Carbs: 5; Protein: 24

Beef In Tomato Marinade

(Prep + Cook Time: 2 hours 15 minutes | Servings: 4)

Ingredients:

- 2 tsp. chili powder
- 1 cup tomatoes; crushed
- 4 beef medallions
- 2 tsp. onion powder
- 2 tbsp. coconut aminos
- 1 jalapeno pepper; chopped
- A pinch of sea salt
- Black pepper to the taste
- 1 tbsp. hot pepper
- 2 tbsp. lime juice

Instructions:

1. In a bowl; mix tomatoes with hot pepper, aminos, chili powder, onion powder, a pinch of salt, black pepper and lime juice and whisk well.
2. Arrange beef medallions in a baking dish, pour the sauce over them and leave them aside for 2 hours.
3. Discard tomato marinade, place beef on preheated grill over medium high heat, cook them for 5 minutes one each side basting them with the marinade.
4. Divide beef medallions on plates, sprinkle jalapeno on top and serve.

Nutrition Facts Per Serving: Calories: 230; Fat: 4; Fiber: 1; Carbs: 3; Protein: 14

Paleo Beef Curry

(Prep + Cook Time: 45 minutes | Servings: 4)

Ingredients:

- 1 tsp. mustard seeds

- 2 tbsp. coconut oil
- 2 curry leaves
- 1 Serrano pepper; chopped
- 1 onion; chopped
- 1 tbsp. garlic; minced
- 1/4 cup water
- 2 tsp. garam masala
- 1 small ginger piece; grated
- 1/4 tsp. chili powder
- 1/2 tsp. turmeric powder
- 1 tsp. coriander powder
- 1 lb. beef; ground
- A pinch of sea salt
- Black pepper to the taste
- 3 carrot; chopped
- 10 oz. canned coconut milk

Instructions:

1. Heat up a pan with the oil over medium high heat, add mustard seeds, stir and toast them for 1 minute.
2. Add Serrano pepper, onion and curry leaves, stir and cook for 5 minutes.
3. Add ginger and garlic, stir and cook for 1 minute.
4. Add beef, a pinch of salt, black pepper, coriander powder, turmeric, chili and garam masala, stir and cook for 10 minutes.
5. Add carrot and 1/4 cup water, stir and cook for 5 minutes more.
6. Add coconut milk, stir well and cook for 15 minutes. Divide curry into bowls and serve.

Nutrition Facts Per Serving: Calories: 260; Fat: 4; Fiber: 5; Carbs: 9; Protein: 14

Paleo Beef Skillet

(Prep + Cook Time: 50 minutes | Servings: 4)

Ingredients:

- 1 lb. beef; ground
- 1 tbsp. parsley flakes
- 2 big tomatoes
- 2 yellow squash; chopped
- 2 green bell peppers; chopped
- 1 yellow onion; chopped
- A pinch of sea salt
- Black pepper to the taste

Instructions:

1. Place tomatoes on a lined baking sheet, place in preheated broiler for 5 minutes, leave them to cool down, peel and roughly chop them.
2. Heat up a pan over medium high heat, add onion and beef, stir and cook for 10 minutes.
3. Add tomatoes, stir and cook for a couple more minutes.
4. Add parsley flakes, black pepper and a pinch of sea salt, stir and cook for 10 minutes more.
5. Add bell pepper pieces and squash ones, stir and cook for 10 minutes. Divide between plates and serve.

Nutrition Facts Per Serving: Calories: 190; Fat: 3; Fiber: 4; Carbs: 6; Protein: 20

Paleo Roasted Lamb

(Prep + Cook Time: 2 hours 40 minutes | Servings: 4)

Ingredients:

- 15 garlic cloves; peeled
- 2 tsp. onion powder
- 6 lamb shanks

- 2 tsp. cumin powder
- 1 cup water
- 3 tsp. oregano; dried
- 1/2 cup olive oil
- A pinch of sea salt
- Black pepper to the taste
- 1/2 cup lemon juice

Instructions:

1. Place garlic cloves in a roasting pan.
2. Add lamb on top, drizzle half of the oil and season with a pinch of salt and black pepper.
3. Also add onion powder and cumin and rub well.
4. Introduce this in the oven at 450 °F and roast for 35 minutes.
5. In a bowl mix the rest of the oil with the water, lemon juice and oregano and whisk very well.
6. Take lamb shanks out of the oven, drizzle this mix, toss to coat well and roast in the oven at 350 °F for 2 hours and 30 minutes. Divide lamb pieces between plates and serve.

Nutrition Facts Per Serving: Calories: 170; Fat: 2; Fiber: 2; Carbs: 4; Protein: 12

Paleo Thai Curry

(Prep + Cook Time: 40 minutes | Servings: 4)

Ingredients:

- 1 yellow onion; chopped
- 3 Thai chilies; chopped
- 2 tbsp. avocado oil
- 1 lb. beef; ground
- 1 small ginger pieces; grated
- 3 garlic cloves; minced
- 1/2 tsp. cumin
- 1/2 tsp. turmeric
- A pinch of sea salt

- Black pepper to the taste
- A pinch of cayenne pepper
- 1 tbsp. red curry paste
- 1 cup tomato sauce
- 1 broccoli head; florets separated
- 1 handful basil; chopped
- 2 tsp. lime juice
- 2 tbsp. coconut aminos

Instructions:

1. Heat up a pan with the oil over medium heat, add chilies and onion, stir and cook for 5 minutes.
2. Add a pinch of salt, ginger, garlic, cumin, turmeric, black pepper, cayenneand beef, stir and cook for 10 minutes.
3. Add broccoli and curry paste, stir and cook for 1 minute more.
4. Add basil, tomato paste and coconut aminos, stir; bring to a simmer, cover, reduce heat to medium-low and cook for 15 minutes. Add lime juice, stir; divide into bowls and serve.

Nutrition Facts Per Serving: Calories: 200; Fat: 3; Fiber: 5; Carbs: 7; Protein: 24

Paleo Beef Patties

(Prep + Cook Time: 35 minutes | Servings: 4)

Ingredients:

- 2 sweet potatoes; boiled and grated
- 1 lb. beef; ground
- 1 cup red onion; chopped
- 2 Serrano peppers; chopped
- 1 small ginger piece; grated
- A handful cilantro; chopped
- 4 garlic cloves; minced
- 1/2 tsp. meat masala

- A pinch of cayenne pepper
- 1/4 tsp. turmeric powder
- Black pepper to the taste
- 1 egg; whisked
- 4 tbsp. almond meal
- 1 cup water
- 5 tbsp. ghee

Instructions:

1. Heat up a pan over medium high heat, add beef, masala, turmeric, black pepper to the taste and cayenne pepper, stir and brown for a few minutes.
2. Add water, stir; cook for 10 minutes more and take off heat.
3. Heat up a pan with 2 tbsp. ghee over medium heat, add Serrano peppers and onion, stir and cook for 2 minutes.
4. Add garlic and ginger, stir and cook for 1 minute more.
5. Add cilantro and the meat mixture, stir well and take off heat.
6. Add grated sweet potatoes, stir well, cool everything down and shape patties from this mix.
7. Put the egg in a bowl and almond meal in another.
8. Dip patties in egg and then in almond meal.
9. Heat up a pan with the rest of the ghee over medium heat, add beef patties, cook them well on one side, flip, cook on the other as well and transfer them to paper towels. Serve them with a side salad.

Nutrition Facts Per Serving: Calories: 180; Fat: 3; Fiber: 3; Carbs: 6; Protein: 15

Special Paleo Beef Dish

(Prep + Cook Time: 45 minutes | Servings: 4)
Ingredients:
- 1 lb. beef; ground

- 1 tsp. cumin seeds
- 1 lb. sweet potatoes; cubed
- 3 tbsp. ghee
- 2 onions; chopped
- 1 small ginger pieces; grated
- 1 Serrano pepper; chopped
- 2 tsp. coriander powder
- 2 tsp. garam masala
- Black pepper to the taste
- 1 cup green peas
- A handful cilantro; chopped

Instructions:

1. Heat up a pan with 2 tbsp. ghee over medium heat, add sweet potato cubes, stir; cook them for 20 minutes and transfer them to a bowl.
2. Heat up the same pan over medium heat, add cumin, stir and brown them for 1 minute. Add Serrano pepper and onion, stir and cook for 4 minutes.
3. Add beef, ginger, coriander, garam masala, cayenne and black pepper, stir and cook for 5 minutes more.
4. Add green peas and sweet potatoes, stir; cook for 5 minutes more, divide between plates and serve with cilantro on top.

Nutrition Facts Per Serving: Calories: 160; Fat: 3; Fiber: 1; Carbs: 5; Protein: 12

Paleo Beef And Cabbage Delight

(Prep + Cook Time: 20 minutes | Servings: 4)

Ingredients:

- 1 onion; chopped
- 1 lb. beef; ground
- 1 napa cabbage head; shredded
- 1 carrot; grated
- A pinch of sea salt

- Black pepper to the taste
- 2 tbsp. coconut oil

Instructions:

1. Heat up a pan with the oil over medium high heat, add onion and beef, stir and brown them for 5 minutes.
2. Add carrots, cabbage, a pinch of salt and black pepper to the taste, stir and cook for 5 minutes more. Divide between plates and serve.

Nutrition Facts Per Serving: Calories: 150; Fat: 1; Fiber: 2; Carbs: 5; Protein: 9

Paleo Slow Cooked Lamb Shanks

(Prep + Cook Time: 4 hours 10 minutes | Servings: 4)

Ingredients:

- 2 big lamb shanks
- A pinch of sea salt
- 1 garlic head; cloves peeled
- 4 tbsp. olive oil
- Juice of 1/2 lemon
- Zest from 1/2 lemon; grated
- 1/2 tsp. oregano; dried

Instructions:

1. Put lamb shanks in your slow cooker, sprinkle a pinch of sea salt, add garlic cloves, cover and cook on High for 4 hours.
2. In a bowl; mix olive oil with lemon juice, lemon zest and oregano and whisk well.
3. Transfer lamb shanks to a cutting board, discard bones, shred meat and divide between plates. Drizzle the lemon dressing on top and serve with a Paleo side salad.

Nutrition Facts Per Serving: Calories: 180; Fat: 2; Fiber: 2; Carbs: 4; Protein: 9

Paleo Thai Lamb Chops

(Prep + Cook Time: 1 hour 15 minutes | Servings: 4)

Ingredients:

- 1/3 cup basil; chopped
- 2 garlic cloves; chopped
- 2 tbsp. Thai green curry paste
- 2 tbsp. avocado oil
- 1 tbsp. gluten free tamari sauce
- 1 small ginger piece; grated
- 2 lbs. lamb chops
- 1 tbsp. coconut oil
- 1 tbsp. coconut aminos

Instructions:

1. In your food processor, mix basil with garlic, curry paste, avocado oil, tamari sauce, aminos and ginger and blend really well.
2. Put lamb chops in a bowl; add basil mix over them, toss well and keep in the fridge for 1 hour.
3. Heat up a pan with the coconut oil over medium high heat, add lamb chops, cook for 2 minutes on each side, introduce pan in the oven and roast lamb at 400 °F for 10 minutes. Serve lamb chops with a side salad.

Nutrition Facts Per Serving: Calories: 170; Fat: 3; Fiber: 2; Carbs: 5; Protein: 14

Greek Beef Bowls

(Prep + Cook Time: 35 minutes | Servings: 4)

Ingredients:

- 1 lb. beef; ground
- 1 tbsp. coconut oil
- 2 garlic cloves; minced
- 1 yellow onion; chopped
- A pinch of sea salt
- Black pepper to the taste
- 1 tbsp. savory; dried
- 1 tbsp. parsley; dried
- 2 tbsp. oregano; dried
- 3 oz. kale; chopped
- 3 oz. endives; chopped
- 1/4 cup kalamata olives; pitted and sliced
- 1/4 cup green olives; pitted and sliced

Instructions:

1. Heat up a pan with the coconut oil over medium high heat, add garlic, onion, a pinch of salt and black pepper, stir and cook for 3 minutes.
2. Add beef, stir and cook for 10 minutes.
3. Add endives, kale, savory, oregano and parsley, stir and cook for 5 minutes more.
4. Add green and kalamata olives, stir; place in preheated broiler and broil for 4 minutes. Divide into bowls and serve.

Nutrition Facts Per Serving: Calories: 367; Fat: 7; Fiber: 4; Carbs: 9; Protein: 30

Steak And Blueberry Sauce

(Prep + Cook Time: 30 minutes | Servings: 4)

Ingredients:

- 1 cup beef stock
- 2 tbsp. shallots; chopped
- 2 garlic cloves; minced
- 1 cup blueberries

- 4 medium flank steaks
- 2 tbsp. ghee
- 1 tsp. thyme; chopped
- A pinch of sea salt
- Black pepper to the taste

Instructions:

1. Heat up a pan with the ghee over medium heat, add shallot and garlic, stir and cook for 4 minutes.
2. Add thyme, stock, a pinch of salt and black pepper, stir; bring to a simmer and cook for 10 minutes.
3. Add blueberries, stir and cook for 2 minutes more
4. Place steaks on preheated grill over medium high heat, cook for 4 minutes son each side and transfer to plates. Drizzle the blueberry sauce on top and serve them.

Nutrition Facts Per Serving: Calories: 170; Fat: 4; Fiber: 3; Carbs: 7; Protein: 15

Paleo Lavender Lamb Chops

(Prep + Cook Time: 2 hours 10 minutes | Servings: 4)

Ingredients:

- 4 lamb chops
- 2 garlic cloves; minced
- 1 tbsp. lavender; chopped
- 2 tbsp. rosemary; chopped
- A pinch of sea salt
- Black pepper to the taste
- 1 tbsp. ghee
- 3 small orange peel; grated

Instructions:

1. In a bowl; mix lamb chops with garlic, lavender, rosemary, orange peel, a pinch of salt and black pepper, rub well and keep in the fridge for 2 hours.

2. Heat up your grill over medium high heat, grease it with the ghee, place lamb chops on it, grill for 5 minutes on each side, divide between plates and serve with a side salad on the side.

Nutrition Facts Per Serving: Calories: 160; Fat: 2; Fiber: 1; Carbs: 4; Protein: 10

Paleo Beef And Brussels Sprouts

(Prep + Cook Time: 22 minutes | Servings: 4)

Ingredients:
- 1 lb. beef; ground
- 1 apple; cored, peeled and chopped
- 1 yellow onion; chopped
- 3 cups Brussels sprouts; shredded
- A pinch of sea salt
- Black pepper to the taste
- 3 tbsp. ghee

Instructions:
1. Heat up a pan with the ghee over medium high heat, add beef, stir and brown for 2 minutes.
2. Add Brussels sprouts, stir and cook for 3 minutes more.
3. Add onion and apple, stir and cook for 5 minutes more.
4. Add a pinch of sea salt and black pepper to the taste, stir; cook for 1 minute more, divide among plates and serve.

Nutrition Facts Per Serving: Calories: 150; Fat: 1; Fiber: 2; Carbs: 3; Protein: 9

Paleo Hamburger Salad

(Prep + Cook Time: 18 minutes | Servings: 4)

Ingredients:
- 2 garlic cloves; minced
- 1 sweet onion; chopped

- 1 tbsp. coconut oil
- 1 lb. beef; ground
- 1 cup cherry tomatoes; chopped
- 1 dill pickle; chopped
- 1 lettuce head; leaves separated and chopped
- A pinch of sea salt
- Black pepper to the taste

For the dressing:
- 2 tbsp. water
- 4 tbsp. mayonnaise
- 2 tbsp. Paleo ketchup
- 1 tbsp. yellow onion; chopped
- 1 tsp. balsamic vinegar
- 1 tbsp. pickle; minced

Instructions:

1. Heat up a pan with the oil over medium heat, add garlic and onion, stir and cook for 2 minutes.
2. Add beef, a pinch of sea salt and black pepper, stir; cook for 8 minutes more and take off heat.
3. In a salad bowl; combine beef mix and with lettuce leaves, 1 dill pickle and cherry tomatoes.
4. In another bowl; mix water with mayo, ketchup, yellow onion, vinegar and 1 tbsp. pickle and whisk well. Drizzle this over salad, toss to coat and serve.

Nutrition Facts Per Serving: Calories: 170; Fat: 3; Fiber: 2; Carbs: 5; Protein: 12

Paleo Beef And Spinach

(Prep + Cook Time: 22 minutes | Servings: 2)

Ingredients:
- 1 big oyster mushroom; chopped
- 2 tbsp. almonds; chopped

- 2 tbsp. ghee
- 4 oz. beef; ground
- 1/2 tsp. chili flakes
- A pinch of sea salt
- White pepper to the taste
- 1 tbsp. capers
- 1/4 cup kalamata olives; pitted
- 1 tbsp. roasted almond butter
- 3 oz. spinach leaves; torn

Instructions:

1. Heat up a pan with the ghee over medium high heat, add mushroom, stir and cook for 3 minutes.
2. Add almonds, stir and cook for 1 minute. Add beef, chili flakes, a pinch of salt and white pepper, stir and cook for 6 minutes.
3. Add almond butter, capers, olives and spinach, stir; cook for a couple more minutes, divide into 2 bowls and serve.

Nutrition Facts Per Serving: Calories: 320; Fat: 2; Fiber: 5; Carbs: 9; Protein: 23

Beef And Veggies

(Prep + Cook Time: 3 hours 10 minutes | Servings: 4)
Ingredients:
- 1 yellow onion; sliced
- 3 garlic cloves; minced
- 1 cup beef stock
- 2 tbsp. coconut oil
- 3 lbs. beef; cut into cubes
- A pinch of sea salt
- Black pepper to the taste
- 8 oz. carrots; sliced
- 8 oz. mushrooms; sliced

- 1 tsp. thyme; chopped

Instructions:

1. Heat up a Dutch oven with 1 tbsp. oil over medium high heat, add beef cubes, season with a pinch of sea salt and black pepper, brown for 2 minutes on each side and transfer to a bowl.
2. Heat up the same Dutch oven over medium heat, add garlic, stir and cook for 2 minutes.
3. Add stock, stir well and heat it up.
4. Return meat to the pot, stir; place in the oven at 250 °F and roast for 3 hours.
5. In a bowl; mix carrots with mushrooms, 1 tbsp. oil, a pinch of sea salt, black pepper to the taste and thyme and stir well.
6. Spread these into a pan, place in the oven at 250 °F and roast them for 15 minutes. Divide beef and juices between plates and serve with roasted veggies on the side.

Nutrition Facts Per Serving: Calories: 200; Fat: 3; Fiber: 4; Carbs: 7; Protein: 20

Paleo Lamb And Eggplant Puree

(Prep + Cook Time: 3 hours 25 minutes | Servings: 4)

Ingredients:
- 4 lamb shoulder chops
- 1 tbsp. ghee
- A pinch of sea salt
- Black pepper to the taste
- 1 cup yellow onion; chopped
- 7 oz. tomato paste
- 2 garlic cloves; minced
- 3 cups water
- 8 oz. white mushrooms; halved

For the eggplant puree:

135

- Juice of 1 lemon
- 1/4 tsp. white pepper
- 2 eggplants
- 4 tbsp. ghee
- A pinch of sea salt

Instructions:

1. Place eggplants on your preheated grill, cookfor 30 minutes, flipping them from time to time, leave them to cool down and peel.
2. In your food processor, mix eggplant flesh with a pinch of salt, white pepper, lemon juice and 4 tbsp. ghee and pulse really well.
3. Spoon eggplant puree on plates and leave aside for now.
4. Heat up a pot with 1 tbsp. ghee, add lamb chops, season with a pinch of salt and black pepper to the taste, stir; brown them for a few minutes on each side and transfer to a plate.
5. Heat up the pot again over medium high heat, add onion, stir and cook for a couple of minutes.
6. Add garlic, stir and cook for 1 minute more.
7. Add mushrooms and tomato paste, stir and cook for 3 minutes more.
8. Add water, return lamb chops, stir; bring to a simmer, cover pot, reduce heat to medium-low heat and cook everything for 2 hours and 20 minutes. Divide lamb chops on eggplant puree and serve.

Nutrition Facts Per Serving: Calories: 200; Fat: 3; Fiber: 3; Carbs: 5; Protein: 10

Easy Beef And Basil

(Prep + Cook Time: 26 minutes | Servings: 4)

Ingredients:

- 6 garlic cloves; minced

- 2 red chilies; chopped
- 1 tbsp. coconut oil
- 1 yellow onion; chopped
- 1½ lbs. beef; ground
- A pinch of sea salt
- Black pepper to the taste
- 3 cups basil; chopped
- 1/2 cup chicken stock
- 2 cups carrot; grated
- 4 tbsp. lime juice
- 2 tbsp. coconut aminos
- 1 tbsp. olive oil
- 1/2 tbsp. honey
- Cauliflower rice for serving

Instructions:

1. Heat up a pan with the coconut oil over medium heat, add onions and a pinch of salt, stir and cook for 4 minutes.
2. Add garlic and chili peppers, stir and cook for 1 minute more.
3. Add beef and black pepper, stir and brown everything for 8 minutes. Add stock and half of the basil, stir and cook for 2 minutes more.
4. In a bowl; mix carrots with 1 tbsp. lime juice, the rest of the basil and the olive oil and stir well.
5. In another bowl; mix coconut aminos with the rest of the lime juice and honey and also stir very well.
6. Divide cauliflower rice on plates,add beef and carrot mix on top and drizzle the honey sauce you've made at the end.

Nutrition Facts Per Serving: Calories: 200; Fat: 3; Fiber: 5; Carbs: 7; Protein: 17

Rosemary Lamb Chops

(Prep + Cook Time: 20 minutes | Servings: 4)

Ingredients:

- 4 lamb chops
- 12 rosemary springs
- 4 garlic cloves; halved
- 1/2 tsp. black peppercorns
- 3 tbsp. avocado oil
- A pinch of sea salt

Instructions:

1. In a bowl; mix lamb chops with a pinch of salt, black peppercorns and oil and massage well.
2. Spread lamb chops on a lined baking sheet and add garlic next to them. Rub rosemary into your palms and add over lamb chops.
3. Introduce everything in preheated broiler over medium high heat for 10 minutes, divide between plates and serve.

Nutrition Facts Per Serving: Calories: 160; Fat: 3; Fiber: 1; Carbs: 2; Protein: 20

Conclusion

If you are worried for lots of health problems, then it is a right time to get rid of processed foods. The foods with high sugar, fat, and salt are not good for your health. These are ruining your health and body; therefore, you should focus on the paleo diet that is a caveman diet. You have to eat real food grown in a natural environment instead of consuming factory and industrial food. These are not good for your health because these are raised with chemicals and preservatives.

The paleo diet will promote the consumption of healthy food items raised in the meadow. You need to follow a particular diet plan with real food and include a regular exercise routine in your life. It will help you to reduce cholesterol, cardiovascular diseases, obesity, diabetes and lots of other health complications.

Part 2

Introduction

In this book you will learn all about the building blocks of the paleo diet so that you can easily implement it in your daily life. As a diet that focuses on a more simplistic way of eating, the paleo diet is optimized to work with your body's genetic profile. This optimization results in your body being more efficient in breaking down and utilizing the foods that you eat so that they are readily available as an energy source. In the following chapters we will cover how to follow the paleo diet plan, how it is different from other diets, the benefits, and some helpful guidelines on what to eat and what to avoid when living a paleo lifestyle. Plus, you will also find 36 delicious, quick and easy paleo recipes for breakfast, lunch and dinner to help you get started today!

Chapter 1: What Is The Paleo Diet?

The paleo diet, also known as the Paleolithic and "Caveman" diet, is an increasingly popular method of dieting today. Not only does this diet plan cater to your body's natural metabolic process, but it also helps to create a balance of your body's chemistry resulting in an overall healthier you. In the following sections, we will take a look at the basics of the paleo diet and demonstrate how this way of eating can be beneficial to you today.

The Basics of the Paleo Diet

The easiest way to understand the paleo diet is to look at the alternate name for it – The Caveman Diet. Essentially it focuses on what we believe our ancestors, or cavemen, would have eaten. As early humans, we consumed what was only readily available to us in a hunting and gathering lifestyle - foods such as meats, nuts, fruits and vegetables. These foods were naturally grown or fed and included no unhealthy additives or preservatives. At that time the early human race was agile. Man was able to outrun predators and chase down prey. Importantly, humans did not suffer from health concerns like diabetes and high cholesterol which are so prevalent today. Over time, however, we have moved against our genetics and ignored how our bodies naturally work. We have progressed from naturally available foods to those designed to have long shelf-lives and which also appeal to chemically driven cravings. The paleo diet takes us away from this artificially focused way of eating and points us back towards foods that our bodies are naturally built to thrive on.

Didn't Cavemen Die Earlier Than We Did?

A commonly asked question when it comes to the paleo diet is – didn't cavemen die earlier than we did? If so, is there not a direct correlation between their shorter lifespan and their diet regime? The average lifespan was indeed shorter than it is today but we must consider the reasons behind this. There is little evidence to suggest that Paleolithic man was dying as a result of heart disease, diabetes, or high cholesterol. Such illnesses were not as common in caveman society in the way that they are today. These medical conditions are directly related to our poor modern diets which focus on excess processed foods laden with colorings, sweeteners, and preservatives. The more prevalent causes of death would have related to the hunting and gathering lifestyle such as being attacked by prey, taking dangerous falls, accidents, and infections. Childbirth among cavemen was precarious. Infancy was dangerous and childhood was difficult. If a caveman lived through these milestones they were more likely to live on to an older age. The advances of modern medicine have also dramatically increased our life expectancy. This is something we take for granted but even the simplest of infections in the Paleolithic times would have contributed to a much shorter lifespan. Rarely would the actual consumption of natural foods have had anything to do with the caveman's cause of death.

So How Does the Paleo Diet Work?

By creating a focus on foods that were naturally available to a Paleolithic society, the paleo diet cuts out hormonally altered, antibiotic filled, and genetically modified foods. It also eliminates artificial preservatives, additives, and food stuffs that are processed. That means no grains, no milk, no refined sugars, and no salty processed foods. Even without these foods, your body will still receive optimal nutrition from naturally occurring foods – fruits, vegetables, nuts, and meats. These foods are more easily broken down by the body so that nutrients can be accessed and converted in to energy. What these foods don't do is provide excess sugars or preservatives that get stored as fat or cause chemical reactions within your body that result in poor health.

Essentially, the paleo diet gives your body the simplest method of fueling itself by offering it the natural foods that it was evolved to be able to easily break down and use.

How Does the Paleo Diet Differ From Other Diets?

The paleo diet is often compared to other diets, particularly the Atkins diet. The reason for this comparison is the belief that both of these diets involve low carbohydrate and high fat intake. The truth is, however, that the paleo diet does not eliminate carbohydrates. Rather, it simply eliminates unhealthy and processed carbohydrates. Eating on the paleo diet, you can get your carbohydrates as well as all other nutrients from natural foods. This differs from diets like the Atkins diet where specific food groups are eliminated (and sometimes reintroduced.) The paleo diet understands that all food groups are necessary for the body to thrive.

Since the foods that you eat on the paleo diet are naturally occurring foods there are no "meal replacement bars" or shakes that contain chemicals, additives and other peculiar supplements. While these other diets rely on the need for "convenience" they also utilize sugars and other unhealthy and unnatural ingredients to make them more palatable.

Another reason that so many people prefer the paleo diet to other diets is that there is no calorie counting, macronutrient ratios to follow, or unpalatable ready-made meals. When eating the paleo diet, you can eat as much as you like of permissible foods. This means that there is no feeling of being starved, no waiting until the next meal and no planning mealtimes and snacks every few hours!

144

Chapter 2: Benefits Of The Paleo Diet

There are more than a few benefits in following the paleo diet. Many of these are obvious, simply due to the nature of the foods being consumed. In the following sections we will cover some of these health benefits, some of which that you may not be familiar with.

Vitamins and Minerals

One of the most significant reasons that the paleo diet is supported by many healthcare providers is because it supports eating whole foods. These fresh foods help to ensure that we eat more of the necessary vitamins and minerals every day. When we don't eat a diet made up of fresh foods we only get a small percentage of the vitamins and minerals that our body requires to remain healthy. Sure, you can pop a multi-vitamin, but not only are those vitamins expensive, but they also use lower quality ingredients. There is also the question of just how useful and advantages multi-vitamins are to your body.

Increased Energy

One of the drawbacks to a diet that is crammed full of foods high in sugar, carbohydrates, additives, and preservatives, is that your body doesn't get the fuel it needs without working hard to get it. Not only that, but the "fuel" that you are providing to your body with this type of diet is quickly burned through, leaving you experiencing what most of us call a "sugar crash." The sugar crash most of us are familiar with happens when foods with high refined sugar content are quickly digested and turned in to glucose (the body's source of energy.) This is like a rapid blast of energy, but the body soon burns through this "fuel" resulting in a crash.

The natural fuel sources eaten on the paleo diet make your body work less to get the energy it needs. These natural foods also provide less "junk" for your body to process. Most importantly, however, the carbohydrates eaten on the paleo diet (almost exclusively obtained from vegetables,) are more slowly digested and are released at a delayed rate in to the blood stream as glucose. What this means is that this "fuel" lasts for longer and doesn't cause rapid spikes in blood sugar.

Increased Satiety

On many different diets, dieters are required to restrict food intake in order to meet calorie goals or nutrient goals for the day. The paleo diet does not impose such restrictions and so paleo dieters can essentially eat as much "paleo friendly" food as they like.

Weight Loss

One of the biggest reasons that people favor the paleo diet is because unlike many other diet plans, it helps one to lose weight quickly, in a natural and healthy way. The elimination of unhealthy processed foods that are high in refined sugars, full of additives, preservatives, saturated fats, and salts, results in incredibly fast weight loss. The best part is that this weight loss is not temporary, as the paleo diet focuses on lifestyle changes.

Better Health and Reduced Risk of Disease

The average paleo dieter has much better health than those on other diets. The reason behind this is the reliance of this diet plan on natural, healthy foods such as fruits and vegetables. These foods provide all of the basic nutrients the body needs to remain healthy and function optimally. In turn, this means that the immune system is working to its full potential and a healthy immune system means less risk of disease. Some of the diseases that can be cured, managed, and prevented on the paleo diet include: high cholesterol, obesity, high blood pressure, diabetes, reduced inflammation, and better control of autoimmune illnesses.

Chapter 3: Eating Guidelines Of The Paleo Diet

In the previous sections, we have talked about the basics of the paleo diet, how it compares to other diets, and the benefits of eating paleo. In this chapter we are going to cover one of the most important things you need to know about eating paleo, what you should and should not eat!

Proteins

The proteins that you eat when following the paleo diet should be lean proteins and they should always be wild caught, free range or grass-fed animals. Some of the proteins that are commonly eaten on the paleo diet are:

- Beef (chuck steak, flank steak, lean veal, and top sirloin steak)
- Poultry white meat
- Lean cuts of pork
- Rabbit
- Goat
- Exotic meats (emu, ostrich, venison, kangaroo)
- Fresh fish
- Poached or boiled egg yolks

Stay away from:
- Fatty cuts of meat
- Processed meats
- Canned fish
- Soy and tofu

- Lentils

- Peanuts

Fats and Oils

Fats and oils tend to confuse many people when it comes to dieting, so we are going to make it simple and give you a basic list of those that are permissible and paleo safe.

- Mono-saturated fats

- Nuts (but not peanuts)

- Avocados and avocado oil

- Toasted sesame oil

- Coconut oil, cream or milk

- Flax seed oil (not for cooking)

- Fish oil

The fats and oils that you want to avoid while eating on the paleo diet include:

- Saturated fats

- Trans fats

- Peanut oil

- Margarine or butter substitutes

- Vegetable oils

- Seed oils

Vegetables

Vegetables are going to make up a good portion of your daily food consumption on the paleo diet. Since there are so many different vegetables that are permissible on this eating plan, we are going to cover just a few and focus on those you should avoid.

- Fiber rich vegetables
- Colorful vegetables
- Vegetables grown above ground
- Root vegetables that are not considered starches
- Colorful fruits (avoid starchy fruits)
- Dry fruits

Vegetables that you want to avoid on the paleo diet include:
- Canned fruits and vegetables
- Sugared or preserved fruits and vegetables
- Pre-prepared fruit and vegetable juices
- Corn
- Legumes
- Beans
- Peas
- Peanuts
- Lentils
- Soy beans

Dairy

Dairy should be avoided or kept to a minimum on the paleo diet. While this is the case, there is a view that butter can stand out as an exception to the likes of milk, cheese and yogurt. Butter, importantly that which is pasture raised or grass-fed, is low in lactose and therefore unlike other dairy products causes little problems to the digestive system or the gut. Avoid diary which is overly processed, as during this procedure it takes away all of the benefits of the healthy fat. Coconut milk is a refreshing substitute for low fat milk. If you still enjoy your small amounts of dairy the overriding and simple rule is to ensure that it is grass-fed, fermented full fat, and pasture raised.

Grains

Agricultural grains and processed foods did not exist in Paleolithic society but were rather developed in later times. Much of these products today contain gluten and lectins which are common factors in causing difficulties and inflammation of the gut. They are also well known as contributory factors to certain heart disease and cancers. Where possible, those following the paleo diet plan should avoid cereals and bread products that contain rye, barley and wheat as these are not generally conducive to the overall wellbeing of the digestive system.

Nuts and Seeds

Nuts and seeds both are a favorite food among people eating on the paleo diet. It is important to know that not all nuts and seeds are permissible, however. Let's take a look first at the nuts and seeds that are permitted on this diet:

- Macadamia nuts

- Almonds

- Pistachios

- Walnuts

- Pine nuts

- Chestnuts

- Pecans

- Hazelnuts
- Brazil nuts
- Cashews
- Pumpkin seeds
- Sunflower seeds
- Flax seeds
- Sesame seeds

Nuts and seeds that you should avoid on the paleo diet include:

- Peanuts
- Salted or seasoned nuts and seeds

Spices

Since the majority of spices are the result of plants, a significant number of spices are permitted on the paleo diet. What you should avoid, however, are spice mixes that contain chemical additives and preservatives or high levels of salt.

What to Drink

As with many diets, the most recommended beverage for those on the paleo diet is just plain water! Also allowed on the paleo diet are:

- Fermented drinks (yes, this includes wine IN MODERATION!)
- Coffee
- Herbal teas
- Green tea

What should you avoid?

- Dairy
- Juices (not including pure fresh juiced vegetables)

- Soda
- Concentrated juice mixes
- Artificially sweetened juices

Chapter 4: 12 Paleo Breakfast Recipes

A great way to get started on the paleo diet is to dig up some recipes to get begin with! In this chapter we will cover twelve of our favorite paleo breakfast recipes for you to try!

Butternut Squash Oatmeal

Servings: 3

Calories: 242

Fat: 6g

Protein: 4.9g

Carbs: 49.9g

Ingredients:

- 1 halved butternut squash seeded
- ¼ cup coconut milk
- ½ tsp. cinnamon
- 1 tbsp. chopped walnuts
- Water

Instructions:

Begin by pre-heating your oven to 350 degrees.

While your oven preheats, add ¼" water to a baking dish that is large enough to fit your butternut squash halves. Place your halves of butternut squash in the water in the dish skin side down.

Once your oven is pre-heated, cook your squash until it is soft – this should take about an hour.

Once cooked, take the squash out of the oven and let it cool.

Once your squash has cooled, scoop out the middle of the squash and put it in a breakfast bowl. Use a fork to mash up the squash and when it has a smooth consistency, add your cinnamon and coconut milk and mix it all together. Once mixed, sprinkle your walnuts on top and serve!

If desired, you can heat this "oatmeal" before eating.

Lemon And Blueberry Muffins

Servings: 12

Calories: 279

Fat: 18.4g

Protein: 8g

Carbs: 25.1g

Ingredients:

- 3 room temperature eggs
- ½ cup melted coconut oil
- ¼ cup coconut sugar
- 1 zested lemon
- 1 tsp. lemon extract
- ¾ tsp. sea salt
- ½ tsp. baking soda
- ¼ tsp. baking powder
- 1 ½ cups almond meal
- 1 cup blueberries

- ½ cup melted coconut butter (for glaze)
- ½ cup raw honey (for glaze)
- 1 juiced lemon (for glaze)

Instructions:

Begin by pre-heating your oven to 350 degrees.

While your oven pre-heats line a 12 cup muffin pan with paper liners.

In a mixing bowl, combine your lemon extract, coconut sugar, lemon zest, coconut oil and eggs and whisk together until well combined.

Over a clean bowl, using a sieve, sieve your baking powder, salt, baking soda together. Next, stir your almond meal in to this dry mixture.

Once your almond meal mixture is well combined, slowly mix in your wet mixture until you get a smooth batter.

Using a silicone spatula, gently fold your blueberries in to the batter.

Next, scoop your batter in to the paper muffin liners, filling each of them ¾ full to leave room for expansion.

Put your muffins in to the oven once it is preheated and bake for 30 minutes or until cooked through.

Once your muffins have cooked through and cooled, take a clean bowl and whisk together your honey, coconut butter and lemon juice for your glaze. When these ingredients are smooth, drizzle it over your cool muffins!

Paleo Pancakes

Servings: 4

Calories: 120

Fat: 7.4g

Protein: 5.7g

Carbs: 8.3g

Ingredients:

- 1 mashed banana
- 3 eggs
- ¼ cup almond flour
- 1 tbsp. almond butter
- 1 tsp. vanilla extract
- ½ tsp. cinnamon
- 1/8 tsp. baking soda
- 1/8 tsp. baking powder
- 1 tsp olive oil

Instructions:

In a mixing bowl, combine your almond butter, banana, almond flour, eggs, vanilla extract, baking soda, cinnamon, and baking powder. Use a whisk to whisk together your ingredients until you get a smooth batter.

Next, add your olive oil to a skillet and heat over medium-high on your stovetop. Once warm, scoop your batter in to your skillet as if you were making traditional pancakes.

Cook your pancakes until you see bubbles in the center, then flip and cook until the other side is browned as well.

Cook all of your pancakes and serve warm with your favorite paleo friendly syrup or topping!

Banana Smoothie

Servings: 1

Calories: 334

Fat: 12.8g

Protein: 3.7g

Carbs: 56g

Ingredients:

- 2 frozen, peeled bananas

- 1 tsp. vanilla extract

- ¼ cup coconut milk

Instructions:

In your blender, combine your vanilla extract and your bananas. Puree these ingredients until they are smooth. Once smooth, add your coconut milk slowly until you get a smoothie consistency. If needed, add more coconut milk.

Pumpkin Breakfast Bread

Servings: 8

Calories: 248

Fat: 13.1g

Protein: 5.8g

Carbs: 28.9g

Ingredients:

- 1 ½ cups almond flour

- ½ cup coconut flour

- 5 tsp. pumpkin pie spice

- 1 ½ tsp. baking soda

- 1 ½ tsp. baking powder

- 1 tsp. sea salt

- 1 can (15 oz.) pumpkin puree (NOT pie filling)

- 4 eggs

- ½ cup maple syrup

- 5 tbsp. melted coconut oil

- 2 tsp. vanilla extract

Instructions:

Begin by pre-heating your oven to 350 degrees. While your oven pre-heats, line a loaf pan with parchment paper.

Now, take a mixing bowl and combine your coconut flour, almond flour, baking soda, pumpkin pie spice, baking powder, and salt. Mix together well using a whisk or your hands.

Now, take another bowl and combine your eggs, pumpkin puree, coconut oil, maple syrup, and vanilla extract. Whisk these ingredients together until blended well and then add in your dry ingredient mixture and whisk together until smooth.

Pour your smooth batter in to your lined loaf pan and then bake in your pre-heated oven for an hour or until cooked through. Allow to cool to warm before eating.

Protein Breakfast Bars

Servings: 20

Calories: 356

Fat: 25.2g

Protein: 12.5g

Carbs: 25.4g

Ingredients:

- 2 cups walnuts

- 1 cup pecans

- 2 cups almonds

- 1 cup pumpkin seeds

- 1 cup dry cranberries

- 1 cup vanilla protein powder of your choice

- ½ cup pitted dates

- ½ cup raisins

- ½ cup coconut flour

- ¼ cup maple syrup

- 3 tbsp. coconut oil

- 1 tbsp. vanilla extract

- 1 ½ tsp. cinnamon

- 1 ½ tsp. molasses

Instructions:

Begin by pre-heating your oven 220 degrees. As your oven is heating, line a baking tray and spread out your pecans and walnuts so that you can bake them.

Once your oven us pre-heated, roast the nuts for 30 minutes until they are fragrant. Remove the nuts from the oven and set aside.

Increase your oven temperature to 230 degrees. As your oven pre-heats again, take a 9" x 13" pan and grease it using coconut butter.

In your blender, combine your pecans, walnuts and your almonds together and pulse until you get a small gravel-like consistency.

Pour this nut mixture in to a mixing bowl and then add in your cranberries, pumpkin seeds, dates, protein powder, raisins, maple syrup, coconut flour, vanilla extract, coconut oil, molasses and cinnamon. Use a silicone spatula to mix these ingredients together well.

Once mixed, scoop these ingredients in to your greased pan. Put your pan in your pre-heated oven and cook for 40 minutes or until browned.

Tropical Raspberry Smoothie

Servings: 2

Calories: 373

Fat: 14.2g

Protein: 3.6g

Carbs: 64.8g

Ingredients:

-       2 bananas cut in to chunks

-       1 cup frozen raspberries

-       2 tbsp. halved pecans

-       1 tbsp. coconut oil

-       1 tbsp. flax seed meal

-       1 pitted date

-       16 fl. oz. water

Instructions:

Put all of your ingredients in to a blender and blend until smooth. Pour in to a glass and serve!

Tropical Fruit Bowl

Servings: 1

Calories: 317

Fat: 16.3g

Protein: 3.3g

Carbs: 45g

Ingredients:

-       1 sliced banana

-       ½ cup frozen peach slices

-       2 tbsp. natural applesauce

- 2 tbsp. water

- 2 tsp. coconut oil

- 1 tbsp. unsweetened shredded coconut (for topping)

- 1 tbsp. sliced almonds (for topping)

- 1 tbsp. raisins (for topping)

Instructions:

In a blender, combine your peaches, ½ your banana, applesauce, coconut oil, and water and blend until you get a smooth consistency.

Pour your blended ingredients in to a bowl and arrange your remaining banana on top of the smoothie. Sprinkle your coconut, raisins, and almonds on top and serve!

Scrambled Eggs And Tomato

Servings: 3

Calories: 264

Fat: 19.7g

Protein: 14.5g

Carbs: 9.2g

Ingredients:

- 2 tbsp. avocado oil

- 6 beaten eggs

- 4 wedged tomatoes

- 2 sliced green onions

Instructions:

In a large skillet, heat 1 tbsp. of your avocado oil on medium heat. Once heated, cook your eggs while stirring with a silicone spatula until they are almost cooked. Once almost cooked, slide your eggs on to a plate.

Now, add the rest of your avocado oil to the skillet and cook your tomatoes until most of the liquid has gone. Now, put your eggs back in the skillet and add in your green onions. Stir these ingredients all together for 45 seconds or so until your eggs are cooked through.

Delicious Dutch Babies

NOTE: This recipe does contain butter!

Servings: 6

Calories: 297

Fat: 25g

Protein: 9.4g

Carbs: 10g

Ingredients:

- 1/3 cup (grass-fed) butter
- 8 eggs
- 1 cup coconut milk
- ¼ cup chestnut flour
- 1/3 cup arrowroot powder
- 1 tsp. lemon extract
- 1g Stevia powder
- ½ tsp. sea salt

Instructions:

Begin by pre-heating your oven to 425 degrees.

As your oven pre-heats, take a 9" x 13" casserole dish and put your butter in to it. Once the oven has pre-heated, put the dish in to the oven so that your butter can melt. When your butter has melted and browned, take the dish out of the oven.

Now, in your blender, pulse your eggs until they are completely smooth. Once smooth, pour in your lemon extract, coconut milk, sea salt, stevia, chestnut flour, and arrowroot powder. Blend these ingredients until they are completely smooth.

Pour your blended arrowroot powder mixture over your melted butter in the casserole dish. Now, put your casserole dish in the oven and cook for 20 minutes or until the middle of your dish is set and the edges are brown.

Eggs In Avocados

Servings: 2

Calories: 248

Fat: 20.9g

Protein: 9g

Carbs: 9.2g

Ingredients:

-	1 halved and pitted avocado
-	2 eggs
-	2 crumbled cooked bacon slices
-	2 tsp. fresh chopped chives

164

- 1 pinch dried parsley

- Sea salt and black pepper to taste

Instructions:

Pre-heat your oven to 425 degrees.

While your oven pre-heats, crack your eggs in to a small mixing bowl.

Now, take a baking dish large enough to fit both halves of your avocado. Set your avocados skin side down and VERY carefully spoon the yolks of your eggs in to the holes in the center of the avocado halves. Fill the rest of the avocado hole with the egg white.

Once you have filled the centers of both of your avocados, sprinkle each egg filled avocado with your parsley, chives, salt and pepper.

When your oven has preheated, bake your egg filled avocados for 15 minutes or until your eggs are cooked through. When cooked completely, put your bacon on top of each avocado half and serve.

Banana Breakfast Smoothie

Servings: 2

Calories: 250

Fat: 12g

Protein: 5.4g

Carbs: 34.9g

Ingredients:

- 2 bananas

- 1 cup frozen peach slices

- 1 tbsp. hemp seeds

- 2 cups water

- 2 tbsp. almond butter

Instructions:

Take out your blender and add in your bananas. On top of your bananas add in your almond butter, sliced peaches, and hemp seeds. Add in your water and puree until you get a completely smooth liquid. Pour in to glasses and serve!

Chapter 5: 12 Paleo Lunch Recipes

Lunch is another important aspect of the paleo diet because it ensures that you eat at regular intervals throughout the day! Let's take a look at twelve of our favorite paleo lunch recipes!

Sweet Potato Curry Soup

Servings: 4

Calories: 340

Fat: 12.8g

Protein: 6.3g

Carbs: 53.3g

Ingredients:

- 3 peeled and diced sweet potatoes
- 2 cups beef broth
- 1 cup unsweetened coconut milk
- 1 minced shallot
- 2 tbsp. maple syrup
- 2 tsp. curry powder
- 1 tsp. sea salt
- 1 tsp. chili powder
- 1 tsp. sweet paprika

Instructions:

In a large pot over medium-high heat, add your sweet potatoes to your beef broth. Cook for around 10 minutes or until all of your sweet potatoes are fork tender.

Once your sweet potatoes are tender, mash them in to the broth with a potato masher.

Once you have mashed your sweet potatoes, add in the rest of your ingredients to the pot and cook for around 10 minutes or until everything is heated through.

When your soup is heated through, take it off the heat and use an immersion blender to smooth it out before serving.

Avocado Chicken Salad Wraps

Servings: 4

Calories: 471

Fat: 25.5g

Protein: 42.7g

Carbs: 21.6g

Ingredients:

-        2 peeled, mashed avocados

-        1 juiced lime

-        2 tbsp. chopped fresh basil

-        ½ tsp. garlic salt

-        ½ tsp. black pepper

-        4 cups chopped cooked chicken

-        ¼ cup raisins or sultanas

-        ¼ cup chopped walnuts

- 2 heads worth of lettuce leaves

Instructions:

In a mixing bowl, combine your avocados with your basil, lime juice, pepper, and garlic salt and using a fork, mash them together.

Once your avocado mixture is well combined and mashed, add in your raisins or sultanas, chicken, and walnuts and stir with a silicone spatula to mix your ingredients together well.

Lay out your lettuce leaves and spoon your chicken salad in to them and roll up.

Egg Muffins

Servings: 12

Calories: 89

Fat: 7.1g

Protein: 5.2g

Carbs: 1.2g

Ingredients:

- 4 chopped slices cooked bacon
- ½ cup diced onion
- ½ cup chopped spinach
- 2 tbsp. olive oil
- ½ cup chopped mushrooms
- 6 beaten eggs
- ¼ cup feta cheese crumbles

169

Instructions:

Begin by pre-heating your oven to 450 degrees.

While your oven pre-heats, line 12 muffin cups with paper liners and grease them with olive oil.

Now, take a skillet and use your fat of choice to grease it. Over medium high heat, heat your skillet and add in your mushrooms, spinach, and onion. Cook these ingredients until your onions are soft. Take the skillet off the heat and set it aside.

In a blender, pulse your onion, spinach, and mushroom mixture until you get a smooth consistency.

Take a mixing bowl and pour your onion mix in to it. Add in your feta cheese, eggs, and bacon and mix together with a silicone spatula until everything is evenly mixed. Pour your mixture in to your muffin cups.

Bake your muffins in your pre-heated oven for 35 minutes or until your muffins are cooked through.

Eggs Marinara

Servings: 4

Calories: 126

Fat: 6.7g

Protein: 7.4g

Carbs: 9g

Ingredients:

-    4 eggs

-    1 cup paleo friendly marinara sauce

- 1 cup water

Instructions:

Begin by pre-heating your oven to 350 degrees.

While your oven pre-heats, heat your 1 cup of water until you get steam, but it is not boiling. Take the steaming water off the heat and pour it in the bottom of a casserole dish.

Now, take four ramekins and add ¼ cup of your marinara sauce in to each ramekin. Crack an egg over each ramekin of marinara and then place the ramekins in to the casserole dish.

Once you have put all four ramekins in to the casserole dish, add more water to make sure that each ramekin is covered up to the halfway point.

When the oven is pre-heated, put your casserole dish in to the oven and bake for 25 minutes or until the eggs are cooked through.

Paleo Beef Stew

This recipe includes butter!

Servings: 6

Calories: 282

Fat: 11.3g

Protein: 23.3g

Carbs: 22g

Ingredients:

- 1 ½ lbs. beef stew meat cubed

- 2 tbsp. butter (grass-fed)

- 1 largely cubed onion
- 1 ½ cups baby carrots
- 1 ½ cups diced potatoes (sweet potatoes if you prefer)
- 3 dry bay leaves
- 1 can (10.75 oz.) tomato soup
- 1 ½ soup cans of water
- 1 tbsp. steak sauce
- 1 packet (1 oz.) of dry onion soup
- ½ tsp. lemon pepper seasoning

Instructions:

In a slow cooker, add your beef and butter. On top of the beef, add in your carrots, onion, potatoes and bay leaves.

In a mixing bowl, combine your steak sauce, water, tomato soup, and onion soup mix. Once they are well mixed, add the liquid ingredients in to the slow cooker and throw your lemon pepper seasoning on top.

Cover your slow cooker and cook on low for 8 to 10 hours until your beef is tender.

Cauliflower Soup

This recipe contains butter!

Servings: 4

Calories: 142

Fat: 7.7g

Protein: 7.9g

Carbs: 12.3g

Ingredients:

- 2 tbsp. butter (grass-fed)
- 1 cup chopped onion
- 5 cups cauliflower chopped
- 2 chopped garlic cloves
- 5 cups low sodium chicken broth
- 1 tsp. sea salt
- ¾ tsp. black pepper
- 1 tsp. white truffle oil

Instructions:

In a large soup pot, melt your butter. Once melted, add in your onions and cook until they are tender.

When your onions are tender, stir your garlic in to the onions and then add your cauliflower. Cook until your cauliflower is softened. Add your chicken broth and salt and pepper in to the pot and stir to mix well.

Cover your pot and allow your soup to simmer for 25 minutes or until your cauliflower is completely fork-tender.

After 25 minutes, take your soup off the stove and use an immersion blender to blend until smooth. Drizzle the top of each bowl with your truffle oil before serving.

Paleo "Pizza"

Servings: 6

Calories: 506

Fat: 27.8g

Protein: 56.5g

Carbs: 5.1g

Ingredients:

- 2 lbs. extra lean ground beef (if possible, grind your own)
- 2 eggs
- ½ cup grated parmesan cheese
- 12 oz. shredded mozzarella cheese
- 1 cup tomato sauce
- 3.5 oz. pepperoni slices
- 1 tbsp. salt
- 1 tsp. caraway seeds
- 1 tsp. oregano
- 1 tsp. garlic salt
- 1 tsp. black pepper
- 1 tsp. red pepper flakes

Instructions:

Begin by pre-heating your oven to 450 degrees.

While your oven pre-heats, take a mixing bowl and add together your caraway seeds, salt, garlic salt, oregano, red pepper flakes, and black pepper. Mix these dry ingredients together well.

In a separate mixing bowl, combine your eggs and beef and use your hands to mix them together thoroughly. Throw your dry ingredients you just mixed in to your meat mixture. Add in your parmesan cheese as well. Mix these ingredients together well.

Grease a 12" x 17" baking pan and press your beef in to the pan as evenly as possible.

Once your oven is pre-heated, bake your dish for 10 minutes or until the meat is not pink anymore. Remove your dish from the oven and drain off any excess grease.

Now, lower the rack in your oven until it is 6" from the heating element and switch on the broiler.

Dust your meat with 1/3 of your mozzarella cheese, then pour your tomato sauce over the cheese. Now dust another 1/3 of your mozzarella cheese over the tomato sauce. On top of the second layer of mozzarella cheese lay out your pepperoni and then cover it with the rest of your mozzarella.

Put your pizza dish in to the oven and broil it until your cheese is golden brown. Remove from the oven, cut and serve!

Paleo Turkey Burgers

Servings: 8

Calories: 206

Fat: 8.6g

Protein: 22.8g

Carbs: 10g

Ingredients:

- 2 lbs. ground turkey

- 1 chopped Granny Smith apple

- ¼ cup chopped mushrooms

- 3 chopped scallions

- 3 tbsp. paleo approved BBQ sauce

- 2 tbsp. spicy mango chutney (store bought)

- 2 tbsp. red pepper jelly

- 2 shakes Worcestershire sauce

- 1 dash sea salt

- 1 dash garlic powder

- Black pepper to taste

- 16 paleo sandwich rounds (not included in nutritional information)

Instructions:

Begin by turning your grill on to medium heat and make sure that the grill grate is oiled just enough to stop your burger from sticking.

While your grill heats, take a large mixing bowl and combine all of your ingredients together. Use your hands to mix everything together well. Once mixed, form 8 patties out of the mixed ingredients and set them on to a plate.

Cook your burger patties on the grill until they are cooked through.

Once cooked, put your turkey burger patty between your paleo sandwich rounds and eat as a burger!

Pecorino Kale Salad

Servings: 4

Calories: 317

Fat: 24.5g

Protein: 9.3g

Carbs: 18g

Ingredients:

- 3 chopped slices pancetta

- 1 can (14 oz.) drained, quartered artichoke hearts

- 1 chopped bunch of kale

- ¼ cup olive oil

- 1 juiced lemon

- 1 tsp. sea salt

- ¾ tsp. black pepper

- ¼ cup grated pecorino cheese

Instructions:

In a skillet, heat 1 tbsp. of your olive oil on medium heat. Once hot, add your pancetta to the pan and cook until it crisps. Once crisp, remove from the pan and set aside on a paper towel to drain.

In the same skillet that you used for the pancetta, cook your artichoke hearts until they are browned. Once browned, put your artichoke hearts aside and turn off your heat.

Now, take a large salad bowl and throw in your kale. Put your artichoke hearts on top and then top those with your pancetta. Sprinkle 3 tbsp. of your olive oil over your salad mixture followed by your lemon juice. Salt and pepper the salad to your taste and then toss it all to combine well.

Before serving, sprinkle your pecorino cheese over the top!

Salmon Burgers

Servings: 4

Calories: 231

Fat: 15.7g

Protein: 19.9g

Carbs: 2.3g

Ingredients:

- 7.5 oz. wild Alaskan salmon cooked and chopped

- ¼ cup almond meal

- 3 eggs

- 2 tbsp. olive oil

- Salt and pepper to taste

- 8 paleo sandwich rounds (not included in nutritional information)

Instructions:

In a bowl, combine your salmon, eggs, almond meal, salt and pepper, and 1 tbsp. olive oil. Use your hands to mix your ingredients together well and then make 4 patties. Set your patties aside.

In a skillet over medium heat, heat 1 tbsp. of your olive oil and cook your patties until they are heated all the way through and browned on the outside.

Serve as is, or serve them between two paleo sandwich rounds if you like!

Turkey Sausage And Broccoli Rabe

Servings: 2

Calories: 688

Fat: 54.6g

Protein: 32.4g

Carbs: 18.7g

Ingredients:

- 4 sliced Italian turkey sausage links

- 3 tbsp. olive oil

- 2 minced garlic cloves

- 2 trimmed bunches broccoli rabe

- Lemon zest to taste

- Dash of red pepper

- Sea salt to taste

- ½ lemon

Instructions:

In a large skillet, heat a little of your olive oil on medium heat – enough to coat the bottom of the skillet.

Once your olive oil is hot, add your sausage slices and cook them until they are brown. Once the sausage is browned, add in your garlic and cook for a minute or so, while stirring. Be careful that your garlic doesn't burn.

Now add in your broccoli rabe and stir to mix. Add lemon zest to your skillet to your taste, and then throw in a dash of red pepper and a dash of sea salt. Mix together to coat your broccoli rabe.

Cook for 15 minutes until your broccoli rabe is wilted. Once wilted, squeeze your lemon over your ingredients in the pan.

Plate your turkey sausage, broccoli rabe mixture and serve.

Paleo Bruschetta

Servings: 4

Calories: 169

Fat: 14.1g

Protein: 2.6g

Carbs: 8.6g

Ingredients:

-     1 drained and chopped can (14 oz.) artichoke hearts

-     2 minced garlic cloves

-     1 tsp. sea salt

-     ½ tsp. black pepper

-     ½ chopped red bell pepper

-     ¼ cup olive oil

-     3 tbsp. chopped fresh basil

-     2 tbsp. chopped red onion

-       1 tbsp. drained capers

Instructions:

In a large mixing bowl, mix together your artichoke hearts with your sea salt, black pepper, and garlic. Make sure to mix thoroughly before adding in your olive oil, red bell pepper, onion, and basil. Stir again gently to mix. Add your capers to the top of your mix and plate!

Chapter 6: 12 Paleo Dinner Recipes

For many people, dinner is the most important meal of the day not only because it provides a significant portion of their nutrition, but also because it allows for family bonding. Below we cover twelve of our favorite paleo dinner recipes that you can make along with your family to encourage healthy family eating!

Paleo Chili

Servings: 4

Calories: 380

Fat: 17.2g

Protein: 33g

Carbs: 26.4g

Ingredients:

- ½ lb. lean spicy ground pork sausage (turkey if preferred)
- 1 lb. ground bison
- 4 minced garlic cloves
- 1 cup chopped red bell pepper
- 1 cup chopped green bell pepper
- 1 cup chopped yellow onion
- 1 ½ tsp. coconut oil
- 1 cup boiling water
- 1 dried chipotle pepper (no stem)
- 1 tbsp. chili powder
- 1 tbsp. cumin
- 1 tsp. oregano
- 1 tsp. unsweet cocoa powder
- 1 tsp. Worcestershire sauce
- 1 can (28 oz.) crushed tomatoes
- 1 ½ tsp sea salt
- ½ tsp. black pepper

Instructions:

Take your boiling water and put your chipotle pepper in to the water and let it soak for 10 minutes or until it is soft. Once soft, take the pepper from the water and mince it finely.

Now, in a large soup pot, melt your coconut oil on medium heat. Once the coconut oil is melted, add in your green bell pepper, onion, and red bell pepper and stir. Let these cook for between 5 to 10 minutes or until your peppers are tender.

Once your peppers are tender, add in your chipotle pepper and your garlic and stir the mixture together. Allow the ingredients to cook for around a minute before stirring in your sausage and bison meat. Allow this to cook for around 10 minutes or until your meat is cooked through.

Once the meat is browned, stir your oregano, chili powder, cumin, cocoa powder, and Worcestershire sauce in to the pot. Mix well and then add in your crushed tomatoes and salt and black pepper. Stir again and let your ingredients come to a boil.

Once your ingredients have come to a boil, turn your heat down to low and let it all simmer for around 10 minutes. Serve!

Paleo Carbonara

Servings: 4

Calories: 428

Fat: 28.7g

Protein: 12.9g

Carbs: 34.4g

Ingredients:

- 1 halved seeded spaghetti squash

- 8 diced slices of bacon

- ¼ cup olive oil

- 1 diced tomato

- 1 tsp. sea salt

- 1 tsp. black pepper
- 4 egg yolks
- 3 sprigs basil

Instructions:

Begin by pre-heating your oven to 400 degrees.

While your oven pre-heats, take a covered baking sheet and place your squash halves peel side down.

Once your oven is pre-heated, bake your squash for 45 minutes or until it is completely tender. When your squash is tender all the way through, shred the inside of the squash in to a bowl using a fork.

Now, take a large skillet and over medium-high heat, heat up your olive oil. Once hot, add in your bacon and cook until it is browned. Once your bacon is cooked, stir in your squash strands. Cook until the squash is completely softened and then add in your tomato and salt and pepper. Stir your ingredients and then take the skillet off the heat.

Add your egg yolks in to your skillet and stir in to the squash without letting it touch the metal of the skillet. Your squash mixture will become creamy in texture. Divide your mix between bowls and throw your basil on top!

Conclusion

I hope this book was able to help to guide you through the ins and outs of the paleo diet. With the information provided in the chapters above, it is my hope that you will not only be able to succeed in losing weight, but that you will also succeed in living a healthier lifestyle.

Now that you have learned all of the basics of the paleo lifestyle, it's time to take the leap and get started! Don't be daunted by this new way of living, it's a better lifestyle choice and a great way to lose weight and stay healthy! Who doesn't want to look fabulous while also making it through cold and flu season without taking a single sick day? Just remember, starting any new diet is a process. You are going to slip up, and you are going to make mistakes, but the important thing is that you keep on going! Believe me, the results of paleo living are definitely worth it!